CLINICAL CASES IN
CONTACT LENSES

CLINICAL CASES IN CONTACT LENSES

Edited by

Ronald K. Watanabe, O.D., F.A.A.O.

Associate Professor of Optometry, Department of Specialty
and Advanced Care, The New England College of Optometry,
Boston; Chief, Cornea and Contact Lens Service,
New England Eye Institute, Boston

With 6 Contributing Authors

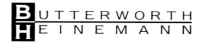

Boston   Oxford   Auckland   Johannesburg   Melbourne   New Delhi

Library of Congress Cataloging-in-Publication Data

Watanabe, Ronald K.
  Clinical cases in contact lenses / Ronald K. Watanabe, with 6 contributing authors.
    p. ; cm.
  Includes bibliographical references and index.
  ISBN 0-7506-7349-4 (pbk. : alk. paper)
  1. Contact lenses—Complications—Case studies. I. Title.
  [DNLM: 1. Contact Lenses—Case Report. WW 355 W324 2002]
  RE977.C6 W28 2002
  617.7'523—dc21
                                                                    2001043144

British Library Cataloguing-in-Publication Data
A catalogue record for this book is available from the British Library.

The publisher offers special discounts on bulk orders of this book.
For information, please contact:

  Manager of Special Sales
  Butterworth–Heinemann
  225 Wildwood Avenue
  Woburn, MA 01801-2041
  Tel: 781-904-2500
  Fax: 781-904-2620

For information on all Butterworth–Heinemann publications available, contact our World Wide Web home page at: http://www.bh.com

10 9 8 7 6 5 4 3 2 1

Printed in the United States of America

This book is dedicated to my parents, Sadao and Terumi, who gave me the ability, the drive, and the love it took to start and finish this project.

Contents

Contributing Authors   xi

Preface   xiii

Acknowledgments   xv

1   Fitting Dilemmas and Complexities

Case 1-1. Low-Riding Rigid Gas-Permeable Contact Lens   3

Case 1-2. Laterally Decentered Rigid Gas-Permeable Contact Lens   9

Case 1-3. High-Riding Rigid Gas-Permeable Contact Lens   15

Case 1-4. Another Low-Riding Rigid Gas-Permeable Contact Lens   19

Case 1-5. Blurry, Uncomfortable Soft Lens   25

Case 1-6. Poor Vision with a Toric Soft Lens   29

Case 1-7. Soft versus Rigid Toric Lenses
Timothy B. Edrington   35

Case 1-8. Unstable Bitoric Rigid Gas-Permeable Lens   39

2   Optical Problems

Case 2-1. Visual Flare, Part 1   47

Case 2-2. Visual Flare, Part 2   51

Case 2-3. Sudden Onset Blur in One Eye   57

Case 2-4. Blurry Vision with Rigid Gas-Permeable Lenses   61

Case 2-5. Blurry Vision with New Rigid Gas-Permeable
Contact Lenses   67

Case 2-6. Double Vision with Soft Toric Lenses   73

Case 2-7. Cloudy Vision   79

Case 2-8. Foggy Vision   83

Case 2-9. Blurry Near Vision
Neil A. Pence   89

Case 2-10. More Problems with Near Vision   95

3   **Fit-Induced Complications**

Case 3-1. Soft Lens Red Eye   101

Case 3-2. Pain with Soft Lens Wear   107

Case 3-3. Soft Lens Discomfort   111

Case 3-4. Redness with Rigid Gas-Permeable Lenses   117

Case 3-5. More Redness with Rigid Gas-Permeable
Lenses   123

Case 3-6. Itchy Soft Lens   127

Case 3-7. Itchy Rigid Gas-Permeable Lens   133

Case 3-8. Soft Lens Discomfort   139

Case 3-9. Routine Soft Lens Wearer   143

Case 3-10. "There's a White Spot on My Eye"   147

Case 3-11. Pain and Redness with Soft Lens Wear   153

Case 3-12. Rigid Gas-Permeable Lens Discomfort   159

Case 3-13. Painful Red Eye with Soft Lens Wear   165

4   **Specialty Contact Lens Fitting Dilemmas**

Case 4-1. Uncomfortable Rigid Gas-Permeable Lens in
Keratoconus
Edward S. Bennett   173

Case 4-2. Bifocal Contact Lens Problem 179

Case 4-3. Difficult Rigid Gas-Permeable Lens Fit
Timothy B. Edrington 185

Case 4-4. Postsurgical Glare 189

Case 4-5. Postsurgical Rigid Gas-Permeable Lens
Intolerance 195

Case 4-6. Uncomfortable Keratoconus Fit 201

Case 4-7. Orthokeratology, Part 1
Marjorie J. Rah 207

Case 4-8. Orthokeratology, Part 2
Harue J. Marsden 215

Case 4-9. Occluder Pupil Lens and a Red Eye
Nadia S. Zalatimo 221

Index 229

Contributing Authors

Edward S. Bennett, O.D., M.S.Ed., F.A.A.O.
Associate Professor and Director of Student Affairs, University of Missouri–St. Louis School of Optometry

Timothy B. Edrington, O.D., M.S., F.A.A.O.
Professor of Cornea and Contact Lens Service, Southern California College of Optometry, Fullerton

Harue J. Marsden, O.D., M.S., F.A.A.O.
Associate Professor of Cornea and Contact Lens Service, Southern California College of Optometry, Fullerton

Neil A. Pence, O.D., F.A.A.O.
Director of Contact Lens Research Clinic, Indiana University School of Optometry, Bloomington

Marjorie J. Rah, O.D., Ph.D., F.A.A.O.
Assistant Professor of Specialty and Advanced Care, The New England College of Optometry, Boston

Ronald K. Watanabe, O.D., F.A.A.O.
Associate Professor of Optometry, Department of Specialty and Advanced Care, The New England College of Optometry, Boston; Chief, Cornea and Contact Lens Service, New England Eye Institute, Boston

Nadia S. Zalatimo, O.D., F.A.A.O.
Chief of Optometry, Manchester Veterans Affairs Medical Center, Manchester, New Hampshire; Assistant Professor of Community Care and Public Health, The New England College of Optometry, Boston

Preface

This collection of clinical cases is meant to provide the clinician and student with a range of contact lens–related complexities and complications that they may encounter in practice. It is by no means representative of every type of contact lens issue that may arise. However, it attempts to address the more common and some not-so-common problems that can be solved with astute examination and analysis skills.

The book is divided into parts emphasizing four areas of contact lens care: fitting dilemmas and complexities, optical problems, fit-induced complications, and specialty contact lens fitting dilemmas. In many of the cases, the problems may fall into two or more of these categories, but they were placed in the parts that seem most appropriate. Therefore, the reader should approach each case individually with no preconceived notion of what the outcome will be.

In writing these cases, the authors may use terminology and abbreviations that are not universal in contact lens practice, particularly outside North America. Ideally, the cases are understandable despite these differences, and the reader can extract the important points of each case.

Every attempt was made to make this book as clinically relevant as possible. By presenting each case with a case history, photo, and pertinent clinical data first, the book allows the reader to figure out the diagnosis and treatment for the case before reading the author's solution. This should stimulate critical thinking on the part of the reader, which is more effective and interesting than passively reading case reports.

The authors hope that the readers will derive benefit from this collection of cases and be better able to manage and care for their contact lens patients.

Ronald K. Watanabe, O.D., F.A.A.O.

Acknowledgments

It was harder than I thought to put together this collection of cases. The book would not have been possible without the help, dedication, and faith of many people. I first thank the editors at Butterworth–Heinemann, who were so patient while they waited for this book to be completed. I also thank the contributing authors, who took the time to compile and write their fabulous cases: Ed Bennett, Tim Edrington, Harue Marsden, Neil Pence, Marjorie Rah, and Nadia Zalatimo. Finally, I thank the love of my life, Nadia, for the support, motivation, and love that carried me to the finish line.

R. K. W.

PART 1

Fitting Dilemmas and Complexities

Low-Riding Rigid Gas-Permeable Contact Lens

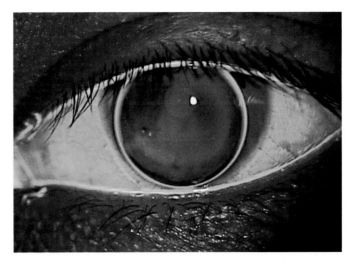

Figure 1-1

History

Patient DE is a 26-year-old Caucasian male who was fit with rigid gas-permeable (RGP) contact lenses (CL) 1 month ago. He presents for his routine 1-month progress evaluation with complaints of mild discomfort and ocular redness that worsen as the day goes on. He reports that he can feel the lenses moving all the time. His wearing time is up to 12 hours per day, but he wants to remove his lenses immediately on returning home from work. However, his vision is very good. He uses Boston Advance Comfort Formula to clean and disinfect his lenses. His ocular and medical histories are unremarkable. He takes no medications and has no allergies.

Symptoms

- Mild discomfort due to excessive lens movement
- Ocular redness that worsens with longer wear times

Clinical Findings

- Visual acuity (VA) with CL:
  OD 20/20
  OS 20/20–
- Keratometry (prior to CL fitting):
  OD 45.50 / 46.75 @ 090
  OS 45.00 / 45.50 @ 080
- Subjective refraction without CL:
  OD +1.00 –1.50 × 180, 20/20
  OS +1.50 –1.00 × 170, 20/20
- Contact lens parameters:
  OD Boston ES / 7.30 / +0.50 / 9.2 / 8.0 / 8.80@0.4 / 9.80@0.2 / 0.20
  OS Boston ES / 7.40 / +1.00 / 9.2 / 8.0 / 8.90@0.4 / 9.90@0.2 / 0.22
- Over-refraction:
  OD Plano –0.25 × 180, 20/20
  OS Plano –0.50 × 170, 20/20
- External exam: Grade 1 interpalpebral conjunctival injection OU
- Biomicroscopy: Grade 2 peripheral corneal desiccation staining OU
- Contact lens fit: Inferiorly positioning RGP lens with rapid vertical movement on blink, steep apical fluorescein pattern with moderate mid-peripheral bearing and minimal peripheral clearance OU (see Figure 1-1)

Based on the clinical data, develop your list of differential diagnoses. Then, determine your final diagnosis and develop your treatment plan.

Differential Diagnosis

- Flat contact lens
- Steep contact lens
- Peripheral corneal desiccation (3 and 9 o'clock staining)
- Primary dry eye
- Solution preservative sensitivity

Diagnosis

Steep contact lens with associated peripheral corneal desiccation

Management

The patient's contact lens parameters were flattened to improve lens positioning and decrease the peripheral corneal desiccation:

- OD Boston ES / 7.40 (45.50) / +1.00 / 9.6 / 8.0 / 8.90@0.4 / 10.90@0.4 / 0.16
- OS Boston ES / 7.50 (45.00) / +1.50 / 9.6 / 8.0 / 9.00@0.4 / 11.00@0.4 / 0.18
- Minus carrier lenticular OU

The patient's discomfort was eliminated, and the peripheral desiccation staining and conjunctival injection were reduced.

Discussion

This case illustrates a fit problem caused primarily by steep, inferiorly positioned rigid contact lenses. RGP lenses fit in this manner can create several problems that can mask the underlying cause.

Comfort

An inferior position is probably the most uncomfortable for a rigid contact lens.[1-4] Every time the lens drops, the wearer feels the edge of the lens hit the lower lid, and with eye movement, the wearer has the sensation of the lens edge rubbing against the lid. In addition, the upper eyelid must traverse the upper edge of the contact lens with every blink. Even with an ideal edge design, the lens is a relatively large obstacle for the upper lid. Thousands of blinks each day may eventually lead to adaptation, but many cannot adapt even with the best edge design.

Blink Characteristics

Because of the discomfort this type of fit creates for the upper eyelid, the normal blink may be inhibited to decrease irritation. This is exacerbated by extended reading, computer work, or other near-point tasks that tend to reduce the blink rate. A constant reduction in blink frequency or completeness results in desiccation of the lens surface, cornea, and conjunctiva. Protein and other films also tend to accumulate on dry lens surfaces, which can lead to further problems with dryness, irritation, and inflammation.

Desiccation

Peripheral corneal desiccation, commonly referred to as *3 and 9 o'clock staining*, can be induced or aggravated by a low-riding rigid lens.[1-4] The tear film overlying the areas adjacent to the lens edge becomes thin and unstable with reduced blinking. In addition, the lens edge, which is very thick compared to the tear film, creates a barrier to the eyelid so that it is unable to rewet the corneal surface with fresh tears when the patient blinks. Unhindered vertical and lateral lens movement can aid in the rewetting of these corneal areas, but a steep-fitting lens does not move as freely, especially in a patient who does not blink often enough. Chronic desiccation can result in stromal and epithelial thinning in these areas.

Injection

Drying of the conjunctiva and peripheral cornea creates a stimulus for the inflammatory response. The earliest manifestation of this is con-junctival injection in the intrapalpebral area. As the cornea becomes dryer, the eyes become more injected. Over time, the inflammatory response can result in infiltration and neovascularization in the desic-cated areas of the cornea.

The key to solving this case is to eliminate the low lens position. Several factors are acting to cause the lens to drop between blinks:

- *Base curve.* A steep lens often drops. Although it may seem logical that steepening the lens further would improve centration, this is not always the case. Often, going toward an alignment fitting rela-tionship helps by increasing the hydrostatic attraction between the contact lens and the cornea.[1,3] *Flatten the base curve by 0.10–0.20 mm.*
- *Lens diameter.* A small lens is less likely to stabilize and remain centered, due to less surface area creating attractive fluid forces with the cornea. In addition, smaller lenses do not attach to the lid as well. To raise the lens into a central or lid-attachment position, a larger lens diameter often helps.[1,2] However, in cases where the lens is dropping and lid attachment cannot be achieved, decreasing lens diameter decreases the lens mass and improves centration.[5,6] *Increase the lens diameter to 9.6 mm.*
- *Center thickness.* A thicker lens has greater mass and more likely will drop, due to a more anterior center of gravity.[1,5] Many new materials provide dimensional strength and stability despite high

Dk values, allowing lenses to be made thinner. *Decrease the center thickness by 0.03 mm.*

- *Edge design.* A plus edge design (thinner at the edge than in the center) is least likely to adhere to the upper lid. To enhance a lid attachment, create a minus edge design via a minus carrier lenticular. This simulates a minus lens edge (thicker at the edge), which is most likely to attach to the upper lid.[7-9] In addition, it allows a decrease in center thickness. *Specify a minus carrier lenticular.*
- *Peripheral curve design.* Flatter peripheral curves increase axial edge lift and improve lens movement toward the limbus. Because the cornea is flatter in the periphery, flatter peripheral curves have less resistance to movement toward the periphery. To enhance lid attachment by allowing less impeded movement to the superior limbus, peripheral curves can be flattened or widened.[7,8] *Flatten the peripheral curve radii by 0.50–1.00 mm.*
- *Eyelid anatomy.* Certain eyelids are not conducive to lid attachments.[1] Ideally, the lid has moderate tightness against the globe and covers 2–3 mm of the superior cornea. If the eyelid is too tight or too loose, the lens will slip out from under the eyelid. If the eyelid is too high, it will not cover enough of the contact lens to create lid attachment. If the upper lid is not likely to attain lid attachment, an interpalpebral fit should be attempted.

Clinical Pearls

- Peripheral corneal desiccation staining may be caused by a low-riding RGP contact lens with poor movement on blink.
- Thick edges and nonoptimal edge lift may exacerbate peripheral desiccation staining.
- Lid attachment may help decrease peripheral desiccation staining by creating better tear film circulation with each blink.

References

1. Mandell RB. *Contact Lens Practice*, 4th ed. Springfield, IL: Charles C Thomas, 1988.
2. Watanabe RK, Byrnes SP. Increasing fitting success with rigid gas-permeable contact lenses. *Practical Optom.* 1996;7(3):100–105.
3. Rakow PL. Managing decentration in rigid lens wearers. *J Ophthal Nursing Tech.* 1998;17(5):199–202.

4. Rakow PL. Spherical rigid gas-permeable contact lenses. *Ophthalmol Clin North Am.* 1996;9(1):31–51.

5. Carney LG, Mainstone JC, Carkeet A, et al. The influence of center of gravity and lens mass on rigid lens dynamics. *CLAO J.* 1996;22(3):195–204.

6. Carney LG, Mainstone JC, Quinn TG, Hill RM. Rigid lens centration: Effects of lens design and material density. *Int Contact Lens Clin.* 1996;23(1):6–11.

7. Sorbara L, Fonn D, Holden BA, Wong R. Centrally fitted versus upper lid-attached rigid gas-permeable lenses. Part I. Design parameters affecting vertical decentration. *Int Contact Lens Clin.* 1996;23(3):99–103.

8. Sorbara L, Fonn D, Holden BA, Wong R. Centrally fitted versus upper lid-attached rigid gas-permeable lenses. Part II. A comparison of the clinical performance. *Int Contact Lens Clin.* 1996;23(4):121–126.

9. Pole JJ, Dominguez A, McNamara N. Lenticular vs. single cut for low plus RGPs: The better design for your patients. *Contact Lens Spectrum.* 1994;9(10):31–32.

Laterally Decentered Rigid Gas-Permeable Contact Lens

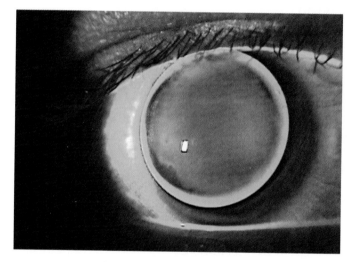

Figure 1-2

History

Patient EM is a 36-year-old Caucasian female who has returned for her initial 2-week progress evaluation. She was fitted with rigid gas-permeable (RGP) contact lenses (CL) 2 weeks earlier. At that time, it was noted that her lenses were somewhat unstable and positioned inferior-temporally most of the time. She was instructed to try to adapt to the lenses. It was felt that, once the initial reflex tearing subsided with increased wear time, the lenses would stabilize. Today, she reports that the lenses still are unstable and uncomfortable. Her vision is good most of the time but blurs as the lenses drop. Her wearing time is up to 6 hours, but she cannot tolerate them any longer than that. She is using Alcon OptiSoak to clean and disinfect her lenses. Her ocular and medical histories are unremarkable. She takes no medications and has no allergies.

Symptoms

- Lens discomfort with RGP lenses
- Fluctuating vision

Clinical Findings

- Visual acuity with CL:
  OD 20/20
  OS 20/20
- Keratometry (prior to CL fitting):
  OD 44.75 / 43.50 @ 090
  OS 44.50 / 43.00 @ 080
- Subjective refraction without CL:
  OD −1.00 −1.00 × 90, 20/20
  OS −2.25 −1.25 × 80, 20/20
- Contact lens parameters:
  OD FluoroPerm 30 / 7.80 / −0.75 / 9.2 / 7.6 / 9.30@0.5 / 11.00@0.3 / 0.18
  OS FluoroPerm 30 / 7.90 / −2.00 / 9.2 / 7.6 / 9.40@0.5 / 11.00@0.3 /0.16
- Over-refraction:
  OD +0.25 −0.25 × 180, 20/20
  OS +0.25 −0.25 × 170, 20/20
- Biomicroscopy: No abnormalities noted OU
- Contact lens fit: Inferior-temporal position, slow rolling movement on blink, apical touch fluorescein pattern with moderate mid-peripheral clearance and moderate peripheral clearance OU (see Figure 1-2)

Based on the clinical data, develop your list of differential diagnoses. Then, determine your final diagnosis and develop your treatment plan.

Differential Diagnoses

- Steep contact lens
- Flat contact lens
- Poor edge design
- Solution preservative sensitivity

Diagnosis

Flat contact lens on an against-the-rule cornea

Management

The patient's lenses were redesigned. The fit was steepened by increasing lens diameter and optic zone to improve the lens-to-cornea relationship, and a minus carrier lenticular edge was added to increase lid attachment. Both changes increased lens stability:

- OD FP30 / 7.80 (43.25) / –0.75 / 9.6 / 8.0 / 9.30@0.5 / 11.00 @0.3 / 0.14
- OS FP30 / 7.90 (42.75) / –2.00 / 9.6 / 8.0 / 9.40@0.5 / 11.00 @0.3 / 0.12
- Minus carrier lenticular OU

The new lenses positioned better with a superior-temporal lid attachment fit. The patient's symptoms decreased, her wearing time increased, and her vision stabilized.

Discussion

This patient's problem is twofold, a flat-fitting lens and an against-the-rule cornea, either of which can cause lens decentration.

Flat-Fitting Lens

A rigid lens with a base curve flatter-than-K tends to decenter toward the flatter peripheral cornea.[1,2] This can be visualized by manually centering a flat lens on a patient's eye and looking at the static fluorescein pattern, which would show central bearing with mid-peripheral and peripheral clearance. A flat lens moves in the direction of least resistance, which is toward the corneal periphery. You may attain lid attachment more easily than with a steeper-than-K lens, but too flat a lens may slip out from under the upper lid, as in this case. Also, a lens that is too flat can distort the cornea and cause spectacle blur.

Against-the-Rule Cornea

Rigid contact lenses use the flat corneal meridian as a fulcrum and move more freely along the steep meridian. For with-the-rule (WTR) corneas, this is ideal because it allows smooth vertical movement and minimal lateral decentration. For against-the-rule (ATR) corneas, lenses tend to move in a nasal-temporal direction, which can be uncomfortable and cause blur for many patients.[1,3]

In this case, the fitting relationship must be reconfigured to prevent lateral decentration. This can be achieved by increasing corneal adherence or lid attachment:

- *Steeper lens design.* Steepening the lens increases corneal adherence, which improves centration and lessens movement.[1] This can be accomplished by decreasing the base curve radius or increasing the optic zone diameter. Both act to increase sagittal depth, which creates greater corneal adherence. *Steepen the base curve radius by 0.10 mm or increase the optic zone diameter by 0.4 mm.*
- *Larger lens diameter.* This aids lid attachment and increases sagittal depth (which steepens the fit).[1] These are opposing forces. While the larger surface area allows the upper eyelid to hold the lens in a superior position more readily, the increased sagittal depth may create a steep fit that causes the lens to drop. If this happens, the base curve or peripheral curves can be flattened to maintain the lid attachment. *Increase the lens diameter by 0.4 mm.*
- *Edge design.* A minus carrier lenticular edge design can increase lid adherence and also allows for thinner center thicknesses for low minus and all plus lenses.[4-6] This can be added if the preceding changes do not solve the problem.
- *Toric back surface.* A final way to improve centration is to increase the lens-to-cornea alignment using toric back surface lenses.[7] These can be designed to match the corneal curves and simulate a spherical lens fit on a spherical cornea. The result is a more stable fit. In this case, this is not recommended because the cornea has too little toricity to stabilize a back toric lens. However, toric peripheral curves can be added to a spherical lens design to improve lens centration. If so, the peripheral curves should be ordered with the same toricity as the cornea. The result is a lens with an oval optic zone and a periphery that more closely aligns with the cornea.

Clinical Pearls

- RGP lenses tend to decenter laterally on against-the-rule corneas.
- Flat-fitting RGP lenses tend to decenter on all corneas.
- RGP fits may be stabilized by steepening the base curve or increasing lens diameter and optic zone.
- RGP lenses may be further stabilized by creating a lid attachment.

References

1. Mandell RB. *Contact Lens Practice*, 4th ed. Springfield, IL: Charles C Thomas, 1988.
2. Watanabe RK, Byrnes SP. Increasing fitting success with rigid gas-permeable contact lenses. *Practical Optom.* 1996;7(3):100–105.
3. Rakow PL. Managing decentration in rigid lens wearers. *J Ophthal Nursing Tech.* 1998;17(5):199–202.
4. Sorbara L, Fonn D, Holden BA, Wong R. Centrally fitted versus upper lid-attached rigid gas-permeable lenses. Part I. Design parameters affecting vertical decentration. *Int Contact Lens Clin.* 1996;23(3):99–103.
5. Sorbara L, Fonn D, Holden BA, Wong R. Centrally fitted versus upper lid-attached rigid gas-permeable lenses. Part II. A comparison of the clinical performance. *Int Contact Lens Clin.* 1996;23(4):121–126.
6. Pole JJ, Dominguez A, McNamara N. Lenticular vs. single cut for low plus RGPs: The better design for your patients. *Contact Lens Spectrum.* 1994;9(10):31–32.
7. Silbert JA. RGP bitorics for high corneal astigmatism. *Optom Today.* 1997;5(5):32–42.

CASE 1-3

High-Riding Rigid Gas-Permeable Contact Lens

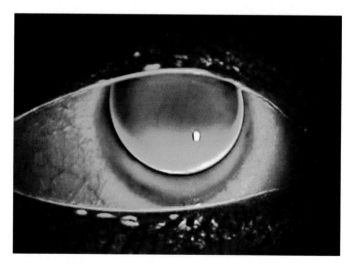

Figure 1-3

History

Patient VP is a 24-year-old Asian male who has been wearing rigid gas-permeable (RGP) contact lenses (CL) for 8 years. He presents for his annual eye examination with complaints of poor comfort with his current contact lenses. He notes that the discomfort increases as the day goes on. His vision is clear. His wearing time is 14–16 hours per day. He uses Allergan Wet-N-Soak Plus to clean and disinfect his lenses. His ocular and medical histories are unremarkable. He takes no medications and has no allergies.

Symptoms

Discomfort with the RGP lenses that increases with longer wear time

Clinical Findings

- Visual acuity with CL:
  OD 20/20
  OS 20/20
- Over-refraction:
  OD Plano sphere, 20/20
  OS Plano –0.50 × 180, 20/20
- Contact lens fit: Superior lens position, minimal movement on blink, apical alignment with mid-peripheral alignment and moderate peripheral clearance, with-the-rule pattern (pattern changes to apical touch with lens centration) (see Figure 1-3)
- Contact lens verification:
  OD 7.75 / –6.75 / 9.4 / 0.11 / unknown RGP material
  OS 7.85 / –6.50 / 9.4 / 0.11 / unknown RGP material
- Keratometry:
  OD 43.50 / 45.25 @ 095, mild distortion
  OS 43.00 / 45.25 @ 085, mild distortion
- Subjective refraction:
  OD –7.00 –2.00 × 005, 20/20–
  OS –7.00 –2.25 × 175, 20/20
- External exam: Grade 1 diffuse conjunctival injection OU
- Biomicroscopy: Grade 1 diffuse conjunctival staining OU

Based on the clinical data, develop your list of differential diagnoses. Then, determine your final diagnosis and develop your treatment plan.

Differential Diagnoses

- Flat fit
- Steep fit
- Warped lens
- Lens flexure
- Hypoxia
- Giant papillary conjunctivitis

Diagnosis

Flat-fitting RGP lenses on a moderately toric cornea

Management

Due to the amount of corneal astigmatism, the patient was refit to an aspheric back surface design RGP lens with a steeper base curve. Although this lens did not align completely with the corneal toricity, it aligned better than the spherical design lens. The new lens centered better and exhibited improved movement. The patient noticed improved comfort. New lens parameters:

- OD Boston 7 Envision / 7.60 / –7.50 / 9.3
- OS Boston 7 Envision / 7.70 / –7.25 / 9.3

The new contact lenses demonstrated good centration, with 2–3 mm movement on blink, minimal apical clearance with mid-peripheral alignment and moderate peripheral clearance. A moderate with-the-rule pattern was still observable.

Discussion

High-riding RGP lenses are often found on moderate to high with-the-rule corneas, especially when the lenses are fit too flat.[1-3] The flat RGP lens tends to want to move toward the flattest part of the cornea, which is the periphery. Also, the direction of least resistance to movement for an RGP lens on a with-the-rule cornea is vertical, so the lens moves either superiorly or inferiorly. Finally, if the upper eyelid tends to grab the RGP lens, it will position and hold it superiorly. Over time, the lens will begin to bind superiorly, and as the post-lens tear film dries due to the lack of lens movement, the lens can adhere and become irritating.[4] Once bound to the cornea, the lens can create corneal distortion as the upper eye lid puts pressure on the lens, resulting in spectacle blur and decreased visual acuity on refraction.

To minimize the chance that the lens will position superiorly, the lens design must be optimized to promote lens centration. On a moderately toric cornea, this is often difficult to achieve. Although a steeper, smaller-diameter lens is ideal for interpalpebral fitting, the smaller diameter often causes the lens to decenter even further on a toric cornea.

This patient also has a lens that is too flat for the corneal curvatures. When a cornea has moderate to high toricity, it cannot be fit on flat-K even though this type of lens aligns well in the flat meridian. Overall, it is too flat for the cornea, and the lens ends up decentering along the steep meridian. A general guideline for toric corneas is to select an initial base curve one quarter to one third the amount of corneal cylinder steeper than the flat K-reading.[1]

Once the optimal base curve has been found, the next step is to select an appropriate lens back surface design. A bitoric design is often ideal, but for a cornea with 2 diopters of toricity, it is not always necessary.[5] In these cases, a spherical or aspheric back surface often suffices.[6] Because the aspheric design is junctionless and more closely matches the corneal eccentricity, it tends to have a greater area of alignment with the cornea than spherical designs. Therefore, an aspheric RGP may perform well on an eye that cannot wear a spherical design. If the aspheric design is also fitting poorly, the bitoric design can be used, as long as the cornea has at least 2 diopters of toricity.

Clinical Pearls

- Flat fitting RGP lenses decenter on the eye.
- RGP lenses decenter superiorly or inferiorly on a with-the-rule cornea.
- Aspheric and toric back surface RGP lenses perform better than spherical lenses on toric corneas.

References

1. Mandell RB. *Contact Lens Practice*, 4th ed. Springfield, IL: Charles C Thomas, 1988.
2. Rakow PL. Managing decentration in rigid lens wearers. *J Ophthal Nursing Tech*. 1998;17(5):199–202.
3. Rakow PL. Spherical rigid gas-permeable contact lenses. *Ophthalmol Clin North Am*. 1996;9(1):31–51.
4. Swarbrick HA, Holden BA. Rigid gas-permeable lens binding: Significance and contributing factors. *Am J Optom Physiol Optics*. 1987;64(11):815–823.
5. Silbert JA. RGP bitorics for high corneal astigmatism. *Optom Today*. 1997;5(5):32–42.
6. Edwards K. A review of rigid lens design. *Contact Lens Ant Eye*. 2000;23:106–111.

Another Low-Riding Rigid Gas-Permeable Contact Lens

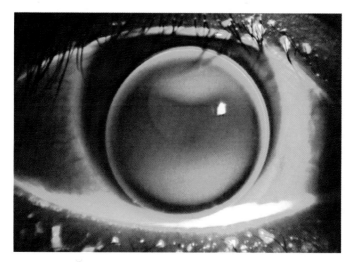

Figure 1-4

History

Patient JT, a 26-year-old Asian male, presents for his 1-week progress evaluation on his new rigid gas-permeable (RGP) contact lenses (CL). This is his first experience with contact lenses, and he would like to wear them full time. He complains of moderate discomfort and feels that the lenses are moving excessively. His vision is unstable as well. His maximum wearing time is 4 hours. He uses the Boston Advance Comfort Formula care system. His ocular and medical histories are unremarkable. He takes no medications and has no allergies. He is a third-year engineering student.

Symptoms

- Discomfort due to excessive movement of RGP lenses
- Unstable vision with contact lenses

Clinical Findings

- VA with CL:
  OD 20/20
  OS 20/20
- Over-refraction:
  OD Plano sphere, 20/20
  OS Plano sphere, 20/20
- Contact lens parameters:
  OD: FluoroPerm 30 / 7.75 / –3.75 / 9.0 / 7.8 / 9.00 @ 0.4 / 11.00 @ 0.2 / 0.14
  OS: FluoroPerm 30 / 7.80 / –3.00 / 9.0 / 7.8 / 9.00 @ 0.4 / 11.00 @ 0.2 / 0.15
- Lens fit assessment: The lenses drop to an inferior position after each blink. Static fluorescein pattern evaluation reveals apical alignment with good peripheral clearance. It appears that the upper lid is squeezing the lens inferiorly after each blink (see Figure 1-4).
- Keratometry:
  OD 43.50 / 44.25 @ 90
  OS 43.00 / 44.00 @ 85
- Subjective refraction:
  OD –3.75 –1.00 × 180, 20/20
  OS –2.75 –1.25 × 175, 20/20
- Biomicroscopy: No abnormalities noted, lid eversion difficult

  Based on the clinical data, develop a list of differential diagnoses for the observed lens behavior. If this movement pattern is unacceptable, redesign the lenses to remedy the problem.

Differential Diagnoses

- Steep fit
- Flat fit
- Tight lids
- Normal adaptation

Diagnosis

Tight upper eyelids

Management

You decide to refit the lenses to achieve better lid attachment, as follows:

- OD: 7.85 / –3.25 / 9.5 / 8.0 / 9.00 @ 0.2 / 10.50 @ 0.35 / 12.00 @ 0.2 / 0.12
- OS: 7.90 / –2.50 / 9.5 / 8.0 / 9.00 @ 0.2 / 10.50 @ 0.35 / 12.00 @ 0.2 / 0.12
- Minus carrier lenticular OU

On dispensing, the new lenses still position inferiorly but now have greater movement and an apical touch pattern with high edge lift. The patient's vision is clear, but he still notes significant discomfort. You decide to refit the lenses to achieve an interpalpebral fit, as follows:

- OD: 7.70 / –4.00 / 8.5 / 7.4 / 9.00 @ 0.35 / 10.00 @ 0.2 / 0.14
- OS: 7.75 / –3.25 / 8.5 / 7.4 / 9.00 @ 0.35 / 10.00 @ 0.2 / 0.14
- Plus edge contour

The lenses demonstrate central position, moderate movement on blink, apical clearance with mid-peripheral bearing, and good peripheral clearance. The patient reports better comfort with these lenses. After 2 weeks of wear, the patient reports clear, stable vision and acceptable comfort that is improving each day. The lens remains centered with good movement, and the corneas show no adverse responses.

Discussion

Low-riding lenses are common in patients who have tight upper eye lids.[1-3] Because greater downward force is exerted onto the lens by the lid, the lens is pushed downward (the "watermelon seed effect"). This is often unavoidable, but if the patient is comfortable and has no ocular problems, it may be acceptable.[4] However, low-riding lenses may cause ocular, vision, or comfort problems.[1-4] If they do, as in this case, we can take two approaches to solving this problem:

1. Lid attachment: To improve a lid attachment, you can do the following:[1,3–5]
   - Flatten base curve and peripheral curves
   - Increase lens diameter
   - Decrease center thickness
   - Add minus carrier lenticular

2. Interpalpebral: This type of fitting technique improves lens centration while reducing the upper lid's interaction with the contact lens when it is in the static position. Movement and stability should be good with each blink. Although this type of fit is thought to be less comfortable initially, the patient can go through a normal adaptation process and achieve comfortable wearing of the lens:[1,3–6]
   - Steepen base curve and peripheral curves
   - Decrease lens diameter
   - Plus edge contour (tapered to a thin, rounded edge apex): This will minimize the upper lid's tendency to push the lens downward by reducing the thickness of the edge. It will also be more comfortable than a thick, round, or minus edge contour.

Either of these solutions will help improve lens centration. Lid attachment is not possible in all patients. Patients who have large palpebral apertures, high upper eyelid positions, or excessively tight upper eyelids may not attain lid attachment.[1,3–5] In these cases, a lens that positions interpalpebrally may perform better. Here, the goal is to maximize corneal adherence while minimizing lid interaction. To attain this, the lens should be fit slightly steep, but not so steep that tear exchange is limited. A mild apical clearance with good mid-peripheral alignment and adequate peripheral clearance should be the fitting goal. In addition, the lens should move with each blink but return to the central cornea soon after the blink cycle has ended. A smaller diameter is usually desirable because it minimizes lens thickness and decreases lens mass, but in cases of larger palpebral apertures, a larger diameter may be needed. In cases of narrow palpebral apertures with tight upper eyelids, a small diameter may be the best solution.

The primary objectives are to optimize patient comfort and vision while minimizing corneal complications. By creating a centered fit, the lens is least likely to create unwanted corneal staining, warping, and binding.

Clinical Pearls

- Low-riding RGP lenses can be made to center better by either improving lid attachment or changing to a smaller, steeper interpalpebral fit.
- Low-riding RGP lenses may create corneal and conjunctival staining or other complications, such as lens adhesion.

References

1. Hom MM, Bruce AS. RGP eyelid geometry. In: Hom MM (ed). *The Manual of Contact Lens Prescribing and Fitting with CD-ROM*, 2nd ed. Boston: Butterworth–Heinemann, 2000.
2. Poland JD. The eyelid's critical role in lens fitting. *Contact Lens Forum*. 1990;15(4):24–28.
3. Rakow PL. Managing decentration in rigid lens wearers. *J Ophthal Nursing Tech*. 1998;17(5):199–202.
4. Mandell RB. Fitting methods and philosophies. In: Mandell RB (ed). *Contact Lens Practice*, 4th ed. Springfield, IL: Charles C Thomas, 1988:204–207.
5. Finnemore V. How the eyelids help and hurt contact lens wear. *Contact Lens Spectrum*. 1994;9(2):26–32.
6. Forst G. The relationship between the eye, eyelid and negative pressure on contact lens movement. *Int Contact Lens Clin*. 1985;12(1):35–40.

Blurry, Uncomfortable Soft Lens

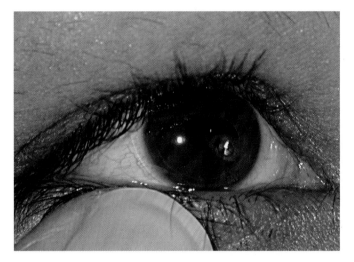

Figure 1-5

History

JC, a 31-year-old Caucasian male, presents for his first soft contact lens progress evaluation. He complains of variable vision and mild lens awareness later in the day. He has built up his wear time to 8 hours per day. He uses the ReNu Multipurpose solution to clean and disinfect his lenses. His ocular and medical histories are unremarkable. He takes no medications and has no allergies.

Symptoms

- Variable vision
- Mild lens awareness later in the day

Clinical Findings

- VA with CL:
  OD 20/25
  OS 20/25+2
- Over-refraction:
  OD Plano –0.25 × 090, 20/25
  OS +0.25 –0.25 × 090, 20/25^{+2}
- Retinoscopy reflex is distorted inferior centrally OU
- Contact lens parameters: OU Biomedics 55 / 8.6 / 14.2 / –3.50
- Contact lens fit: Central position, 0.5 mm movement on blink, no lag on upgaze, minimal movement on push-up (see Figure 1-5)
- Biomicroscopy: All structures clear and healthy OU
- Keratometry:
  OD 43.75 / 44.50 @ 090
  OS 44.25 / 44.50 @ 090
- Subjective refraction:
  OD –3.50 –0.25 × 090, 20/20
  OS –3.25 –0.25 × 090, 20/20

Based on the clinical data, develop your list of differential diagnoses. Then, determine your final diagnosis and develop your treatment plan.

Differential Diagnoses

- Uncorrected astigmatism
- Defective lens optics
- Steep-fitting lens
- Flat-fitting lens
- Dry eye

Diagnosis

Steep-fitting lens

Management

The patient was refit with a lens that has a flatter base curve to improve lens draping and visual acuity:

Biomedics 55 / 8.9 / 14.2 / –3.50 OU

The patient's visual acuity improved to a sharp 20/20 in each eye. The flatter base curve also increased movement, which resulted in increased comfort throughout the day. He was able to attain a wear time up to 14 hours per day.

Discussion

This patient's symptoms were created by a soft lens with too steep a base curve. Even though the base curve is much flatter than K, if the peripheral cornea and sclera are flatter than normal, the lens may fit too tightly. Tight fitting lenses may result in poor comfort and vision.[1-3] The poor comfort is due to decreased lens movement, which results in poor tear exchange, lens binding, and hypoxia. Over time, these factors can lead to further corneal complications, such as acute red eyes and infiltrates. It is important to detect these problems at early follow-up visits to head off more serious complications. In soft lens wearers, staining with sodium fluorescein is often not done for fear that the lenses will be stained. However, it is an important test that can help detect early tight lens–induced changes. For example, changes that are very difficult or impossible to detect without the aid of fluorescein include limbal compression rings, peripheral corneal staining, and peripheral furrow staining.[4] After instillation, fluorescein can be irrigated from the tears with saline solution prior to reinserting the contact lenses. An alternative is to use high-molecular-weight fluorescein, which will not stain soft contact lenses.

Poor vision is sometimes induced by steep soft lenses.[1-3] Because the lenses cannot drape the cornea completely, they attempt to vault the cornea, like a steep-fitting rigid contact lens. However, unlike a rigid lens, a soft lens cannot maintain its shape, and it collapses in the center. The result is a distorted central zone that blurs the patient's vision. Blinking often smooths the soft lens for a short time, during which the patient will observe clearer vision. Diagnostically, you can detect a steep-fitting soft lens by performing over-retinoscopy or over-keratometry.[1-3] The retinoscopy reflex will be dark or distorted in the central or inferior-central portion of the pupil, which is caused by the light rays being scattered in the distorted zone. This may clear on vigorous blinking. On over-keratometry, the mires will be slightly blurry but clear following a blink. Either positive test indicates the need for a flatter base curve.

Even if a patient does not complain on follow-up visits, if the lens appears to be fitting too tightly for any of the preceding reasons, it is important to refit to a flatter base curve to head off future potential tight lens complications.

Clinical Pearls

- Steep-fitting soft lenses may cause discomfort later in the day.
- Steep-fitting soft lenses may cause blurry vision.
- Steep-fitting soft lenses may be detected by retinoscopy or keratometry.

References

1. Mandell RB. Hydrogel lenses with spherical surfaces. In: Mandell RB (ed). *Contact Lens Practice*, 4th ed. Springfield, IL: Charles C Thomas, 1988:544–550.
2. Gasson A, Lloyd M. Soft (hydrogel) lens fitting. In: Philips AJ, Speedwell L (eds). *Contact Lenses*, 4th ed. Oxford, England: Butterworth–Heinemann, 1997:379–380.
3. Guillon M. Basic contact lens fitting. In: Ruben M, Guillon M (eds). *Contact Lens Practice*. London: Chapman and Hall, 1994:599–601.
4. Davis LJ, Lebow KA. Noninfectious corneal staining. In: Silbert JA (ed). *Anterior Segment Complications of Contact Lens Wear*, 2nd ed. Boston: Butterworth–Heinemann, 2000:82–89.

CASE 1-6

Poor Vision with a Toric Soft Lens

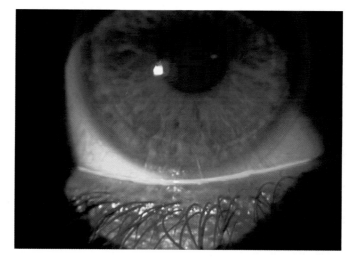

Figure 1-6

History

Patient DS, a 38-year-old Caucasian female, presents with complaints of unstable vision in her right eye. She reports no problems in her left eye. She is a toric soft contact lens (CL) wearer for 3 years. She states that she never had a problem with her vision until she tore her right lens and ordered a replacement 1 month ago. Ever since then, her right eye has been unable to achieve stable, clear vision, despite two lens reorders. She notes that her visual acuity is clear for long periods, followed by stretches of blurry vision later in the day. At that point, manually rotating the lens clears her vision.

She is here to get a second opinion because her previous optometrist told her that her vision is clear and he can do nothing more. Rigid gas-permeable (RGP) lenses were discussed, but she rejected that option. Her average wearing time is 12 hours per day. She uses AOSept to clean and disinfect her lenses. Her ocular and medical histories are unremarkable. She takes multivitamins and has no allergies.

Symptoms

Unstable vision OD with toric soft lens, especially later in the day

Clinical Findings

- VA with contact lenses:
  OD 20/20–
  OS 20/20
- Current wearing time is 3 hours, and she reports that her vision currently is clear
- Over-refraction:
  OD +0.25 –0.50 × 140, 20/20
  OS Plano sphere, 20/20
- Keratometry (after CL removal):
  OD 43.25 / 43.50 @ 090, mires clear
  OS 43.50 / 43.75 @ 080, mires clear
- Subjective refraction without CL:
  OD –2.00 –1.75 × 180, 20/20
  OS –2.25 –1.50 × 170, 20/20
- Contact lens parameters:
  OD: Optima Toric / 8.6 / –2.00 –1.75 × 10 / 14.0
  OS: Optima Toric / 8.6 / –2.25 –1.25 × 170 / 14.0
- Biomicroscopy: No abnormalities noted OU
- Contact lens fit: Central position, 0.5 mm movement on blink, 1 mm lag movement, toric lens markings at 6:00 OD and OS, slow rotation with blinks OD, stable rotation OS (see Figure 1-6)

Based on the clinical data, develop your list of differential diagnoses. Then, determine your final diagnosis and develop your treatment plan.

Differential Diagnoses

- Unstable toric lens rotation
- Steep-fitting lens
- Flat-fitting lens

- Incorrect lens power
- Surface deposits
- Refractive shift OD

Diagnosis

Unstable toric lens rotation

Management

The patient's symptoms suggest a lens that starts out fitting well but later tightens such that the lens rotates and remains off axis. Loosening the fit may alleviate symptoms by preventing the lens from tightening up off axis. New contact lens parameters:

OD Optima Toric / 8.9 / –2.00 –1.75 × 010 / 14.0

If she reports similar symptoms with this new lens, a refit to a soft toric lens with larger diameter or increased prism ballast, or to an RGP lens, would be indicated.

Discussion

Soft toric contact lens fitting can be frustrating because of the difficulty in obtaining clear, stable vision in some patients. The lack of precision in fit characteristics that are sometimes encountered can be further exacerbated by imprecision in lens manufacturing. However, soft toric lens manufacturing has improved considerably to where accuracy and reproducibility generally are very good. Factors that contribute to blurry or unstable vision include the following[1]:

- Inaccurate axis location
- Excessive rotational movement on blink or eye movement
- Slow return to static position after blink
- Flat fit (poor stability of movement and rotation)
- Steep fit (poor draping)

Each of these factors must be ruled out to determine the actual cause of the blurry vision:

- *Inaccurate axis location.* This can be due to rotation of the lens on the eye, inaccurate marking of the lens by the manufacturer, or inaccurate assessment of rotation.[1-4] Because it is very difficult to accurately verify the soft toric lens cylinder axis in office, other possible causes of axis inaccuracy must be ruled out. Rotation can be assessed in the slit lamp by several methods: reticule with protractor, slit beam rotation (on slit lamps with rotational markings), or estimation using lens markings or clock hours. The first two methods are more accurate, although an experienced observer can accurately determine rotation by estimation. A laterally decentered lens must be carefully assessed because the indicator marks on the lens are laterally displaced as well, giving the appearance that the lens is rotated when it is not. Once the amount of rotation is determined, it can be used to adjust the lens axis so that it aligns with the cylinder axis of the eye. LARS or cross-cylinder calculations (via calculators) can be used to determine the final lens axis.[5]

- *Excessive rotation.* Some patients' upper eyelids cause a soft toric lens to rotate on blinks because they move obliquely to the axis of the cylinder power or the prism ballast. In these cases, the patient may notice transient blur, especially as the cylinder power becomes higher.[1–4,6] Tightening the fit by steepening the base curve or increasing lens diameter helps reduce rotation. Increasing the prism ballast by switching to a different lens brand also may help. Finally, refitting to a lens brand with more uniform meridional lens thickness may reduce blink-induced rotation.
- *Slow post-blink return.* Transient lens rotation is often tolerated by patients as long as the lens returns to its static position quickly. Lenses fit too tightly may cause a slow return, which causes noticeable blur.[1,2] Although tighter-fitting soft toric lenses often improve rotational stability, the base curve should not be made so steep that the lens cannot restabilize quickly. Also, complications induced by tight lenses must be detected early and avoided.
- *Flat fit.* Too flat a base curve results in a lens that has less stable movement and rotation.[1,2,4,6] The patient may also note discomfort from excessive movement or edge lift. A loose or unstable lens should be reordered with a steeper base curve or larger diameter.
- *Steep fit.* In addition to causing a slow post-blink return, a steep fit may cause blur via poor draping that results in distortion of the central portion of the lens.[1,2] Blinking may improve clarity but only transiently. A distorted retinoscopy reflex that clears with blinks will help diagnose this problem. Refitting to a flatter base curve helps alleviate this problem.

Clinical Pearls

- A soft toric lens that is fit too steeply may result in the lens tightening up off axis, with resulting blurry vision.
- A blurry retinoscopy reflex also may point to a steep fitting soft lens.
- Flattening the base curve of a soft toric lens will eliminate blurry vision in a steep-fitting lens by allowing it to drape better on the corneal surface.

References

1. Mandell RB. Hydrogel lenses for astigmatism. In: Mandell RB (ed). *Contact Lens Practice*, 4th ed. Springfield, IL: Charles C Thomas, 1988:659–680.
2. Watanabe RK. Managing the astigmat with contact lenses. *Contact Lens Spectrum*. 1999;14(8):42–47.
3. Lindsay RG. Troubleshooting toric soft lenses. *Contact Lens Spectrum*. 2000;15(9):27–33.
4. Becherer PD. Toric lenses, then and now, some timeless pearls. *Eyequest*. 1991;1(1):14.
5. Lindsay RG, Bruce AS, Brennan NA, Pianta MJ. Determining axis misalignment and power errors of toric soft lenses. *Int Contact Lens Clin*. 1997;24(3):101–106.
6. Tomlinson A, Ridder WH, Watanabe R. Blink-induced variations in visual performance with toric soft contact lenses. *Optom Vis Sci*. 1994;71(9):545–549.

Soft versus Rigid Toric Lenses
Timothy B. Edrington

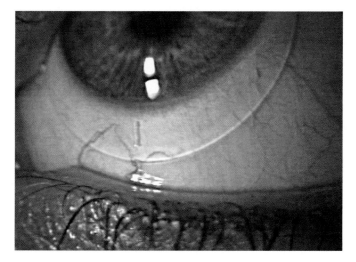

Figure 1-7

History

Patient JS is a 27-year-old female presenting with a chief complaint of poor vision through her habitual toric soft contact lenses (CL). The vision through her spectacles is excellent. Both were prescribed to her approximately 9 months ago. At the time of her initial toric soft contact lens fitting, three different pairs were ordered and dispensed. In each case, the lenses did not provide her with crisp vision comparable to her spectacles. JS wears her lenses on a daily wear basis with a maximum wearing time of 14 hours per day. The patient is compliant with the care of her lenses.

Symptoms

Blurred vision with the soft toric lenses

Clinical Findings

- Visual acuity with habitual toric soft contact lenses:
  OD 20/20–
  OS 20/25+
- Habitual CL fit:
  OD 1.0 mm movement on blink, lag and sag; prism base marking at 5:30 o'clock, lens rotation stable on blink
  OS 1.5 mm movement on blink, lag and sag; prism base marking at 6:00 o'clock, lens rotation not stable (20° on blink) (see Figure 1-7)
- Keratometry:
  OD 41.87 @ 170 / 45.12 @ 080; no mire distortion
  OS 42.25 @ 005 / 44.75 @ 095; no mire distortion
- Manifest refraction:
  OD $-0.75 -2.75 \times 165$, $20/15^{-2/6}$
  OS $-1.50 -2.25 \times 010$, $20/15^{-1/6}$
- Biomicroscopy: OU central cornea clear, no staining, mild ($<\frac{1}{2}$ mm) perilimbal vascularization

Based on the clinical data, develop your list of differential diagnoses. Then, determine your final diagnosis and develop your treatment plan.

Differential Diagnoses

- Flat soft contact lens causing cylinder misalignment due to excessive rotation during or after a blink
- Cylinder misalignment due to prescribing wrong axis
- Crisp vision not afforded by toric soft contact lens due to cylinder component in excess of sphere component

Diagnosis

The vision afforded JS is not acceptable with toric soft contact lenses. This probably is due to the patient having a low tolerance for blur. Refitting into different parameters or designs of soft torics is unlikely to resolve her symptoms due to her rejection of three previous pairs of soft toric contact lenses. JS is a candidate for rigid contact lenses, spectacle-only wear, or part-time wear of soft torics.

Management

After discussing the advantages and disadvantages of the various contact lens options, a rigid contact lens fitting was performed. Spherical rigid gas-permeable (RGP) diagnostic lenses are positioned inferiorly. It was decided to prescribe the following bitoric RGPs empirically:

$$OD \frac{44.12D / -2.50 D}{41.37 D / -.25 D} / 9.2 / 7.6 / 8.80 / 12.00 / 0.2 / 0.19 / \#1 \text{ blue}$$
/ Dk = 30

$$OS \frac{43.75 D / - 2.75 D}{41.75 D / - 1.00 D} / 9.2 / 7.6 / 8.80 / 12.00 / 0.2 / 0.17 / \#1 \text{ blue}$$
/ Dk = 30

Patient JS was refitted into RGP contact lenses to enhance the crispness and consistency of her vision. After adaptation, JS reported excellent vision through the RGPs and no noticeable spectacle blur after lens removal. Follow-up visits revealed an alignment fitting relationship, minimal over-refraction, and no corneal staining.

Discussion

The patient is a compound myopic astigmat. Soft toric contact lenses did not provide her with optimal vision. Perhaps, refitting the patient into a different base curve, power, axis, or manufacturer's toric soft contact lens may have alleviated the symptom of blurred vision. Decreased vision through a soft toric soft lens generally is caused by cylinder axis mislocation or instability of axis rotation. If the lens rotates more than 10° on a blink or if the lens does not return to relatively the same position after each blink, suspect a flat-fitting lens and consider refitting with a steeper base curve or a larger overall diameter. The larger the cylinder correction, the more critical is rotation stability.[1]

The decision to prescribe bitoric, instead of spherical, rigid contact lenses was based on the positioning of the spherical diagnostic rigid contact lenses on the cornea. Consider prescribing toric back surface rigid lens designs when the corneal toricity, as assessed by keratometry, videokeratography, or fluorescein pattern, is equal to or exceeds 1.50 diopters.[2,3] If the corneal toricity is 3.00 diopters or more, a toric back surface design is indicated.

Clinical Pearls

- If practical, allow soft toric contact lenses to settle or equilibrate for a minimum of 20 minutes prior to evaluating the lens fit, rotation, and rotation stability.
- If a patient is not satisfied with the vision through his or her toric soft contact lenses, consider fitting a spherical or toric RGP.
- Bitoric RGPs should be considered for patients with 1.50 D or more of corneal toricity. Even though a spherical RGP might provide good comfort and vision, corneal molding or induced corneal distortion tends to be reduced with a bitoric design. Therefore, the patient will experience less spectacle blur.

References

1. Snyder C. A review and discussion of crossed cylinder effects and over-refractions with toric soft contact lenses. *Int Contact Lens Clin.* 1989;16(4):113–118.
2. Sarver MD, Kame RT, Williams CE. A bitoric gas-permeable hard contact lens with spherical power effect. *J Am Optom Assoc.* 1985;56(3):184–189.
3. Edrington TB. Rigid gas-permeable lenses for astigmatism. In: Hom MM (ed). *Manual of Contact Lens Prescribing and Fitting with CD-ROM*, 2nd ed. Boston: Butterworth–Heinemann, 2000:143–165.

Unstable Bitoric Rigid Gas-Permeable Lens

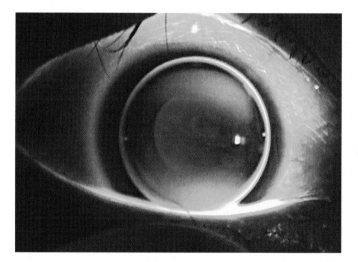

Figure 1-8

History

Patient MA, a 32-year-old Hispanic female, presents for a progress evaluation of her new rigid gas-permeable (RGP) bitoric contact lenses (CL). She reports having difficulty adapting to her lenses, which move a lot and give her unstable vision. She has been able to wear her contact lenses only up to 5 hours per day. She uses Boston Advance Comfort Formula care system to clean and disinfect her lenses. Her ocular and medical histories are unremarkable. She is taking no medications and has no allergies. Her occupation is accountant for a legal firm.

Symptoms

- Excessive lens movement
- Unstable vision with contact lenses

Clinical Findings

- VA with CL:
  OD 20/30
  OS 20/30
- Over-refraction:
  OD Plano –0.50 × 180, 20/30+
  OS +0.25 –0.75 × 175, 20/25
- Keratometry:
  OD 41.25 / 45.50 @ 090
  OS 41.50 / 46.00 @ 085
- Subjective refraction:
  OD +1.25 –4.75 × 180, 20/25
  OS +1.50 –5.25 × 175, 20/25
- External exam: Unremarkable OU
- Biomicroscopy: No abnormalities noted OU
- Contact lens parameters: Boston ES,

  OD $\dfrac{41.25 / +1.25}{44.50 / -2.00}$ / 9.0 / 7.6 / 9.7 @ 0.5 / 11.0 @ 0.2 / 0.20

  OS $\dfrac{41.50 / +1.50}{45.00 / -2.00}$ / 9.0 / 7.6 / 9.7 @ 0.5 / 11.0 @ 0.2 / 0.20

- Contact lens fit: Inferior position, 3 mm movement on blink, apical alignment with high inferior peripheral clearance, moderate with-the-rule fluorescein pattern OU (see Figure 1-8)

  Based on the clinical data, develop your list of differential diagnoses. Then, determine your final diagnosis and develop your treatment plan.

Differential Diagnoses

- Steep fit
- Flat fit
- Undercorrection of corneal cylinder
- RGP intolerance
- Normal RGP adaptation

Diagnosis

Undercorrection of corneal cylinder resulting in a loose fit

Management

The fluorescein pattern indicates that there is too little corneal toricity to stabilize the lens. Specifying toric peripheral curves further stabilizes the fit. In addition, the uncorrected astigmatism in the over-refraction can be eliminated with a power adjustment. New bitoric lens parameters:

Boston ES

$$\text{OD } \frac{41.25 \, / +1.25}{45.00 \, / -3.00} \; / \, 9.0 \, / \, 7.6 \, / \, \frac{9.7}{9.9} \; @ \, 0.5 \, / \, \frac{11.7}{11.0} \; @ \, 0.2 \, / \, 0.20$$

$$\text{OS } \frac{41.50 \, / +1.75}{45.50 \, / -3.00} \; / \, 9.0 \, / \, 7.6 \, / \, \frac{9.7}{9.0} \; @ \, 0.5 \, / \, \frac{11.7}{11.0} \; @ \, 0.2 \, / \, 0.20$$

With these adjustments, the lenses attained a more central position with less movement on blink. The fluorescein pattern showed apical alignment with a slight with-the-rule pattern and uniform peripheral clearance OU. The patient was able to adapt to the new lenses more easily and reached a maximum of 12 hours of wear time.

Discussion

The bitoric RGP contact lens is a wonderful option for moderate to high astigmats.[1-5] It has all the advantages of RGP lenses, including sharp vision and fewer ocular complications, and allows moderate to high astigmats to wear rigid contact lenses that are stable during the course of normal wear. It may also minimize the corneal molding that would be induced by a poor fitting relationship, such as when a spherical lens is fit to a highly toric cornea. However, the bitoric lens can be challenging to fit, especially when not used frequently.

Base Curve Selection

For a with-the-rule cornea, the bitoric lens base curves should be selected to simulate the fitting of a spherical RGP on a near-spherical cornea.[1-5] This results in a lens with a base curve toricity less than the corneal toricity by 0.50–1.25 D in most cases, which is optimal because the lens attains a stable central to superior-central position more easily. To do so, the flat meridian is fit on-K or 0.25 D flatter-than-K, while the steep meridian is fit flatter-than-K by one quarter of the amount of corneal toricity.[1-4]

In this case, although the base curve radii were ordered according to these guidelines, the lens ended up undercorrecting the corneal toricity. The moderate toricity in the fluorescein pattern is evidence of this: the horizontal flat meridian has good alignment, but the vertical steep meridian has a flat-fitting relationship. This indicates that a steeper vertical meridian should be ordered. This change reduces the amount of toricity in the fluorescein pattern, leaving a slight with-the-rule pattern.

Peripheral Curves: Spherical or Toric?

The peripheral curve system is essential in the proper behavior of a rigid lens on the eye. Since most (although not all) astigmats have toric peripheral as well as central corneas, the lens should be designed with toric peripheral curves for better peripheral alignment.[3] This minimizes the problem of excessive edge lift in the steep meridian and peripheral binding in the flat meridian. By specifying peripheral curve radii that are toric by the same amount as the base curve radii, the contact lens has uniform peripheral clearance. This will allow the contact lens to better attain a central position while minimizing peripheral corneal complications where the edge lift is not optimal.

Power Determination: The Optical Cross

The optics of the bitoric lens can be somewhat confusing. Unlike spectacle or soft toric contact lens prescriptions, bitoric lens powers are specified for each major meridian. The optical cross is the best way to avoid confusing the powers in each meridian. When there is a spherocylindrical over-refraction, it must also be placed on an optical cross to be able to determine the final prescription. Once the proper powers are placed on the cross, it is simple to sum each meridian.[1-5]

For the right eye, the new contact lens powers in each major meridian are determined independently, as shown in Table 1-8. Through careful fluorescein pattern assessment and optical cross calculations, bitoric RGP contact lens fitting problems can be solved.

Table 1-8   Optical Cross Calculation for the
             Right Lens

	Horizontal	*Vertical*
Lens power	+1.25	–2.00
BC change	Plano	–0.50 (steeper BC, must add minus)
Over-refraction	Plano	–0.50
Total	+1.25	–3.00

Clinical Pearls

- Bitoric RGP lenses should simulate the fit of a spherical RGP on a low with-the-rule cornea.
- Undercorrecting the corneal cylinder may result in an unstable or loose fitting relationship.
- Use of toric peripheral curves may add stability to the bitoric lens fit.
- Use optical crosses to determine the final prescription for bitoric RGP lenses.

References

1. Sarver MD, Mandell RB. Toric lenses. In: Mandell RB (ed). *Contact Lens Practice*, 4th ed. Springfield, IL: Charles C Thomas, 1988:292–305.
2. Sarver MD, Kame RT, Williams CE. A bitoric gas-permeable hard contact lens with spherical power effect. *J Am Optom Assoc.* 1985;56(3):184–189.
3. Edrington TB. Rigid gas-permeable lenses for astigmatism. In: Hom MM (ed). *Manual of Contact Lens Prescribing and Fitting with CD-ROM*, 2nd ed. Boston: Butterworth–Heinemann, 2000:143–165.
4. Silbert JA. RGP bitorics for high corneal astigmatism. *Optom Today.* 1997;5(5):32–42.
5. Watanabe RK. Managing the astigmat with contact lenses. *Contact Lens Spectrum.* 1999;14(8):42–47.

PART 2

Optical Problems

Visual Flare, Part 1

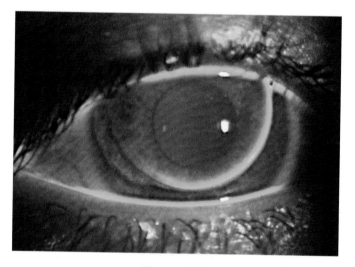

Figure 2-1

History

A 26-year-old Caucasian male presents for his first progress evaluation with complaints of flare with his new rigid gas-permeable (RGP) contact lenses (CL). This is his first experience wearing contact lenses. He notices the flare at night and indoors but does not notice it in daylight. He is otherwise satisfied with his contact lenses. His wearing time is up to 8 hours per day, but he removes the lenses as soon as he gets home from work because of the flare. He uses Boston Advance Comfort Formula to clean and disinfect his lenses. His ocular and medical histories are unremarkable. He takes no medications and has no allergies.

Symptoms

Visual flare with the RGP lenses, especially under low light conditions

Clinical Data

- Entering visual acuity with CL:
  OD 20/20
  OS 20/20
- CL specifications:
  OD 7.85 / –2.25 / 9.0 / 7.8 / Polycon II
  OS 7.90 / –2.50 / 9.0 / 7.8 / Polycon II
- Over-refraction:
  OD Plano sphere, 20/20
  OS +0.25 sphere, 20/20
- CL fit assessment: Superior-central position, 2 mm movement on blink, lid attachment, apical alignment with moderate peripheral clearance OU (see Figure 2-1)
- Keratometry:
  OD 43.00 / 43.75 @ 090
  OS 43.00 / 44.25 @ 090
- Subjective refraction:
  OD –2.25 –0.75 × 180, 20/20
  OS –2.50 –1.25 × 180, 20/20
- Gross external exam: Eyes appear white and quiet OU
- Biomicroscopy: All structures appear clear and healthy OU

Develop your list of differential diagnoses. Then, based on the clinical data, determine your final diagnosis. Based on your diagnosis, develop your treatment plan.

Differential Diagnoses

- Optic zone diameter too small
- Lens decentration
- Incomplete adaptation
- Poor blending of optic zone junction
- Overminused

Diagnosis

Optic zone diameter is too small

Management

The lens diameter and optic zone diameter were increased to decrease the patient's symptoms of flare:

OD 7.90 / –2.00 / 9.4 / 8.2 / Paraperm O$_2$
OS 7.95 / –2.00 / 9.4 / 8.2 / Paraperm O$_2$

The patient noticed markedly reduced flare, although it remained present to a small degree. He was educated about the reasons for the flare and explained that it diminishes with adaptation. He increased his wear time gradually to 14 hours and reported that the flare was noticeable only under very dark conditions.

Discussion

A rigid gas-permeable contact lens with a small optic zone often causes flare.[1-4] From the photo of the lens fit, it is apparent that this contact lens has an optic zone too small for the patient's pupil size. This is even more evident considering that the pupil size in an ocular photograph very likely is smaller than it would be under dark lighting conditions. Since this patient's complaints occur under dimmer illumination conditions, it is important to measure the pupil size in a dark room. Also, because he is a young Caucasian male with blue irises, he is more likely to have larger pupils and therefore notice visual flare from the optic zone junction. The patient will be able to ignore some amount of flare as he adapts. However, in this case, the optic zone diameter should be increased.

Another consideration is the position of the lens. Because the lens rides superiorly in a lid attachment position, the optic zone is shifted upward. This brings the inferior edge of the optic zone toward the pupil, which makes the flare even more noticeable. Therefore, it is helpful, in this case, to improve lens centration to further decrease the flare. The two simplest changes to improve centration are increasing lens diameter and steepening the base curve.[1-5] Since we already increased the optic zone diameter, it makes sense to also increase the lens diameter by the same amount. In general, a 0.3–0.4 mm increase in both diameters is sufficient. This change improves centration by covering more of the cornea and also by steepening the fit. Any increase in the optic zone diameter, and to a lesser extent the overall diameter of an RGP lens, steepens the fitting relationship. This is visible during fluorescein pattern assessment. Too steep a fitting relationship can be offset by flattening the base curve radius.

Other possible lens changes include increasing the blend of the optic zone–secondary curve junction or changing to a junctionless aspheric back surface design.[1-3] In this case, it is obvious that the primary cause of the patient's flare is the small optic zone diameter. However, in cases where the optic zone is larger than the pupil, blending the optic zone helps diminish flare. In extreme cases, an aspheric back surface design can be used as well, but the flare will remain present to some degree because of the changing refracting power in the lens periphery as the back surface flattens.[1]

The patient's symptom is much reduced by changing the overall diameter and optic zone diameter of the lens. Although he still notices some flare in dark environments, it is tolerable. Patient education on the cause of his visual flare also decreases the patient's concerns. It is good practice to present visual flare as a potential observation for all new RGP wearers, particularly during the adaptation stages. By presenting this potential symptom prior to the lens fitting, the patient is more likely to accept it and adapt to it.

Clinical Pearls

- Visual flare can be caused by a large pupil, small optic zone, or lens decentration.
- Visual flare is common early in RGP adaptation.
- Patient education prior to fitting RGP lenses helps reduce complaints of visual flare after initial dispensing.

References

1. Hodur NR, Gandolfi B, Wojciechowski S. Flare with rigid contact lenses. *Contact Lens Forum.* 1986;11(3):48–49.
2. Hom MM. Rigid lens design and fitting. In: Hom MM (ed). *Manual of Contact Lens Prescribing and Fitting with CD-ROM*, 2nd ed. Boston: Butterworth–Heinemann, 2000:77–103.
3. Rakow PL. Spherical rigid gas-permeable contact lenses. *Ophthalmol Clin North Am.* 1996; 9(1):31–51.
4. Josephson JE, Caffery BE, Rosenthal P, et al. Symptomatology and aftercare. In: Ruben M, Guillon M (eds). *Contact Lens Practice.* London: Chapman and Hall, 1994:565.
5. Theodoroff CD, Lowther GE. Quantitative effect of optic zone diameter changes on rigid gas-permeable lens movement and centration. *Int Contact Lens Clin.* 1990;17(2):92–95.

Visual Flare, Part 2

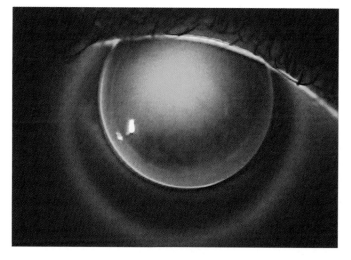

Figure 2-2

History

A 49-year-old Caucasian male presents for his first progress evaluation on his new aspheric multifocal rigid gas-permeable (RGP) contact lenses (CL). He feels that he is adjusting to his new lenses well but is bothered by his night vision. At night, he notices lots of flare and is not comfortable driving with his lenses. He has no visual problems during the day. He also is adjusting well to the comfort of the lenses. He wears his lenses a maximum of 10 hours per day. He uses Optimum Care System to clean and disinfect his lenses. His ocular history is significant for blepharitis. His medical history is unremarkable. He takes no medications and has no allergies.

Symptoms

Visual flare with aspheric multifocal RGP lenses, especially at night

Clinical Data

- Entering visual acuity with CL at distance:
  OD 20/20–
  OS 20/25
- Entering visual acuity with CL at near:
  OD J-1
  OS J-1+
- CL specifications:
  OD 7.60 / –4.00 / 9.5 / Blanchard Essential Series II / Boston ES
  OS 7.70 / –3.50 / 9.5 / Blanchard Essential Series II / Boston ES
- Fit assessment: Superior central position, 2 mm movement on blink, apical clearance, mid-peripheral bearing, wide peripheral clearance OU (see Figure 2-2)
- Over-refraction:
  OD Plano sphere, 20/20– at distance, J-1 at near
  OS –0.50 sphere, 20/20– at distance, J-1 at near
- Keratometry:
  OD 43.25 / 43.75 @ 090
  OS 42.75 / 43.50 @ 090
- Subjective refraction:
  OD –3.00 –0.50 × 180, 20/20
  OS –3.00 –0.75 × 180, 20/20
  Add +1.75
- Gross external exam: Eyes appear white and quiet OU
- Biomicroscopy: Grade 1 blepharitis OU, otherwise all structures appear clear and healthy OU

Develop your list of differential diagnoses. Then, based on the clinical data, determine your final diagnosis. Based on your diagnosis, develop your treatment plan.

Differential Diagnoses

- Optic zone diameter is too small
- Lens decentration
- Incomplete adaptation
- Overminused
- Aspheric optics causing optical distortion

Diagnosis

Aspheric optics causing the patient's optical distortion

Management

Because of the nature of aspheric multifocal RGP lenses, flare is to be expected in dim light, particularly in new wearers. Because the lenses seemed to be fitting acceptably and this patient was a new lens wearer, he was advised to continue to wear the lenses. He was also advised to remove the lenses and wear spectacles when driving at night.

Discussion

Aspheric multifocal RGP contact lenses have unique optical surfaces that create a progressively changing power from the center to the edge of the optic zone, so that the center of the lens has the most minus power while the periphery has the most plus power.[1-5] This progressive power change provides the patient with multiple focal lengths to enable focusing on objects at different distances. Although this is a benefit for the presbyopic patient, it creates potential visual disturbances.[1-5] These visual disturbances are created by the light rays refracting through the different optical powers in the optic zone all falling on the retina at the same time. Some of the light rays will be in focus while others will not. The result is some amount of visual confusion and blur. The successful aspheric multifocal RGP wearer ignores the unfocused light rays and sees those in focus.

The amount of defocused light incident on the retina depends on the asphericity of the lens surface and the pupil size. The greater the eccentricity (e-value) of the lens surface, the greater is the differential in optical power between the center and edge of the optic zone. A greater eccentricity therefore results in a greater add power but creates more blur than a lower eccentricity lens surface.[1-6] A large pupil allows light traveling through the entire optic zone to enter the eye. A small pupil limits peripheral light rays, resulting in less defocused light reaching the retina. Therefore, the greater the eccentricity (add power) of the lens and the greater the pupil diameter, the more likely it is that the patient will notice problems with distance vision, such as flare.[1-5]

This patient's complaints occurred primarily at night. We can presume that the patient's pupils are larger at night, which would explain why the patient noticed this symptom only then. With single-vision RGP lenses, we can adjust zone diameters to try to decrease the flare.

With multifocals, we lack this luxury. We must therefore minimize flare with good lens positioning and educate the patient on the reasons for these symptoms. We must also advise the patients about wearing times, possibly limiting lens wear to daytime hours.

To improve lens centration, the base curve can be steepened. However, steepening a lens that is already steep centrally would probably result in poor tear exchange, debris entrapment, lens adhesion, and greater corneal distortion. A larger diameter may result in better centration but may also create more lid attachment, which would pull the lens even further upward. This is because as aspheric lenses are made larger, edge lift increases, resulting in greater lid interaction.[1-5]

Because this patient is a new lens wearer who is adapting reasonably well and because aspheric lenses have more limitations on parameter changes, it was decided to keep the patient in the same lenses, provide him with a thorough explanation on the cause of the flare, and recommend that he wear his glasses for night driving. He agreed and was very pleased with his contact lenses at subsequent follow-up visits.

Clinical Pearls

- Aspheric multifocal RGP contact lenses can create flare due to the progressive nature of the optics.
- Fewer options for parameter changes are available with specialty designs, such as aspheric multifocals.
- Patient education is important in decreasing complaints.

References

1. Edwards K. Contact lens problem-solving: Bifocal contact lenses. *Optician*. 1999;218(5721):26–30.
2. Hansen DW. Rigid bifocal contact lenses. *Optom Clin*. 1994;4(1):103–119.
3. Lebow KA. Contemporary RGP bifocals: Fitting and follow-up. *Eyequest*. 1992;2(5):34–46.
4. Watanabe RK. Presbyopia: Contact lenses 2000. *Contact Lens Spectrum*. 2000;15(5):41–47.

5. Schatz S. Improve visual performance with an aspheric multifocal. *Contact Lens Spectrum.* 2000;15(8):37–39.
6. Hodur NR, Gandolfi B, Wojciechowski S. Flare with rigid contact lenses. *Contact Lens Forum.* 1986;11(3):48–49.

Sudden Onset Blur in One Eye

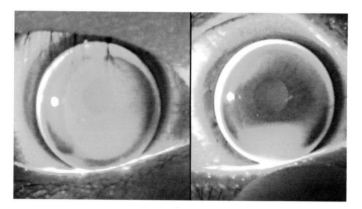

Figure 2-3

History

A 19-year-old Caucasian male presents at his first rigid gas-permeable (RGP) contact lens (CL) follow-up visit with complaints of sudden-onset blurry vision in his right eye only that began 2 days earlier. He was dispensed a new pair of RGP lenses 1 week prior. At that visit, visual acuity was good in each eye. He also notes some discomfort and is discouraged about the lenses, although he knows that he has to adapt to the lenses over the course of 2 or 3 weeks. His current maximum wear time is about 6 hours per day. He is using Boston Advance Comfort Formula Care System. His ocular and medical histories are unremarkable. He takes no medications and has seasonal allergies.

Symptoms

- Sudden onset blur OD with new RGP contact lenses
- Discomfort with new RGP contact lenses

Clinical Data

- Entering visual acuity with CL:
  OD 20/40
  OS 20/20
- Over-refraction:
  OD –1.00 sphere, 20/20
  OS +1.00 sphere, 20/20
- CL specifications:
  OD 7.67 / –3.25 / 9.2 / 8.0 / 9.20 @ 0.4 / 10.20 @ 0.2 / 0.15 / Boston ES
  OS 7.58 / –2.75 / 9.2 / 8.0 / 9.10 @ 0.4 / 10.10 @ 0.2 / 0.l5 / Boston ES
- Fit assessment:
  OD Centered, blink movement 1 mm, apical clearance, mid-peripheral bearing, moderate peripheral clearance
  OS Superior temporal, blink movement 2 mm, apical touch, mid-peripheral clearance, moderate peripheral clearance (see Figure 2-3)
- Keratometry (from previous visit):
  OD 44.00 / 45.25 @ 090
  OS 44.50 / 45.75 @ 090
- Subjective refraction (from previous visit):
  OD –3.25 –1.50 × 180, 20/20
  OS –2.75 –1.50 × 180, 20/20
- Gross external exam: Eyes appear white and quiet OU
- Biomicroscopy: All structures appear clear and healthy OU

Develop your list of differential diagnoses. Then, based on the clinical data, determine your final diagnosis. Based on your diagnosis, develop your treatment plan.

Differential Diagnoses

- Right lens underminused
- Defective lens (wrong power or base curve)
- Warped lens
- Switched lenses
- Myopia progression

Diagnosis

The patient has switched the lenses

Management

The lenses were verified and found to be switched. A dot was placed on the right lens. The patient was educated on lens switches and rescheduled for his next follow-up visit.

Discussion

An examination of the patient's keratometry and refraction data shows that the effective powers of the two RGP lenses are 1.00 D different (OD is flatter with more minus, OS is steeper with less minus). Therefore, because the patient's lenses had been switched, the correction for each eye shifted by 1.00 D. Because the right eye wears a steeper, less minus lens, it was effectively underminused, causing distance blur. The left eye was overminused by the same amount, but because the patient is young, he could accommodate through the extra minus and see clearly.

Observation of the lens fit is also consistent with a lens switch. Because the right eye wears a steeper lens, it has more central clearance and perhaps centers better on the eye. The left eye has a flatter fit with apical touch and more decentration. Final confirmation of a lens switch is made by verifying the base curves and lens powers.

Prevention of lens switches is important in preventing corneal and refractive changes over time.[1,2] Poorly aligning lenses are more likely to cause corneal distortion and spectacle blur. Long-term wearing of poorly fitting lenses may lead to permanent corneal warpage. This is more likely with lower Dk RGP materials. Refractive findings for patients with long-term corneal distortion include changes in astigmatism and decreased best-corrected visual acuity. Corneal topography is also helpful in diagnosing changes in corneal curvature.

Prevention of future lens switches can be ensured by first educating the patients to check their vision after lens insertion. A monocular check with a distant target will let the patient know immediately if the lenses are on the wrong eyes. Another strategy to prevent future switches is to have the RGP laboratory put a black dot at the edge of the right lens. The patient then knows which lens is which before insertion. However, the black dot often rubs off with daily cleaning, especially when using abrasive cleaners such as Boston Cleaner. A final strategy to help the patient is to order two different lens colors: green for the right eye, blue for the left eye. This foolproof method is readily accepted by all but light blue irised patients.

The other differential diagnoses can be easily ruled out by the over-refraction (OR).[1-3] If the patient were underminused in the right eye, the left eye would not have a plus OR nor would the fluorescein pattern change. Defective lens optics would not be correctable to 20/20 with an OR. A defective base curve would change the OR in one eye only. A warped lens would be correctable with a spherocylindrical OR at best, and the best-corrected visual acuity may not be achievable with a warped lens. Myopia progression of 1.00 D is not expected in 1 week.

Clinical Pearls

- Over-refraction and fluorescein pattern assessment are critical to determine visual problems due to lens switching.
- Patient education is important to prevent future lens switches.
- Small dots or different color lenses will help prevent future lens switches.

References

1. Mandell RB. Symptomatology and refitting. In: Mandell RB (ed). *Contact Lens Practice*, 4th ed. Springfield, IL: Charles C Thomas, 1988:411.
2. Josephson JE, Caffery BE, Rosenthal P, et al. Symptomatology and aftercare. In: Ruben M, Guillon M (eds). *Contact Lens Practice*. London: Chapman and Hall, 1994:564–565.
3. McMonnies CW. After-care symptoms, signs and management. In: Philips AJ, Speedwell L. *Contact Lenses*, 4th ed. Oxford, England: Butterworth–Heinemann, 1997:634–635.

Blurry Vision with Rigid Gas-Permeable Lenses

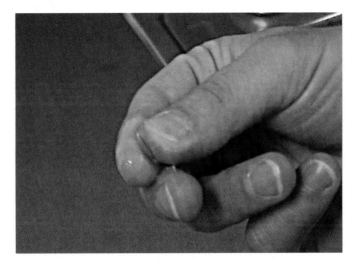

Figure 2-4

History

HG is a 41-year-old Caucasian male accountant. He presents for his annual eye exam with complaints of blurry vision with his contact lenses (CL), especially at near. He reports that this has been a gradual change he has noticed over the past 2–3 months. He bought a pair of +1.50 D drug store readers to wear over his contact lenses, which seems to clear up his vision. He has no complaints about lens comfort and can wear his lenses 14 hours a day. His current right lens is 6 months old, and his left lens is 2 years old. He uses the Boston Original care system to clean and disinfect his lenses. He has a history of rigid contact lens wear for 20 years. His ocular history is unremarkable. His medical history is significant for hypertension, for which he takes propanolol. He has no allergies.

Symptoms

Blurry vision at near with CL

Clinical Data

- Visual acuity with CL at distance:
  OD 20/25
  OS 20/30
- Visual acuity with CL at near:
  OD 20/30
  OS 20/50
- Lens parameters:
  OD FluoroPerm 60 / 7.60 / –1.00 / 9.2 / 8.0 / 9.10 @ 0.4 / 11.00 @ 0.2 / 0.16
  OS FluoroPerm 60 / 7.60 / –1.50 / 9.2 / 8.0 / 9.10 @ 0.4 / 11.00 @ 0.2 / 0.16
- Over-refraction:
  OD +0.50 sphere, 20/20 at distance and near
  OS +1.25 sphere, 20/20 at distance and near
- Lens fit: OU centered, 2 mm movement on blink, mild apical touch, moderate mid-peripheral clearance, good lid attachment
- Keratometry:
  OD 44.75 / 45.50 @ 090
  OS 44.50 / 45.00 @ 090
- Subjective refraction:
  OD –1.25 –0.75 × 180, 20/20
  OS –1.50 –0.50 × 010, 20/20
  No add required, NRA +2.50, PRA –0.75
  Refraction unchanged from previous exam
- External exam: All structures appear white and quiet OU
- Biomicroscopy: Minimal 3 and 9 o'clock staining OU, otherwise unremarkable OU

Develop your list of differential diagnoses. Then, based on the clinical data, determine your final diagnosis. Based on your diagnosis, develop your treatment plan.

Differential Diagnoses

- Lens switch
- Lens flexure
- Overminused
- Altered lens parameters
- Hyperopic refractive shift

Diagnosis

Altered lens parameters have altered

Management

Because the patient's refraction had not changed since the previous visit, the change in over-refraction was puzzling. The lenses were verified as follows:

OD 7.60 / –1.50 / 9.2 / 8.0 / 0.13
OS 7.60 / –2.75 / 9.2 / 8.0 / 0.11

Further questioning revealed that the patient cleans his lenses vigorously between his thumb and forefinger with Boston Cleaner (see Figure 2-4). In addition, he cleans the lenses for at least 1 minute to make sure they are clean. It was determined that he had rubbed the lenses so much that he added minus power to the lenses. Also, the left lens had a greater power change because the right lens had been replaced recently.

The patient was advised of the parameter changes. A new pair of lenses was reordered with the original parameters. Boston Advance Comfort Formula was prescribed, and the patient was educated on proper daily cleaning technique.

Discussion

Although rigid gas-permeable (RGP) materials are very durable, they can be modified if enough pressure is applied.[1-5] In the office, modification tools can be used to change the power, polish the lens surfaces, change the edge shape, and change peripheral curves. At home, patients can also alter lens parameters if an abrasive cleaner is used with heavy finger pressure. Boston Original Cleaner was formulated with abrasive particles to remove hard protein deposits from silicone acrylate RGP materials. This cleaner is often too abrasive for softer RGP materials, such as higher Dk fluorosilicone acrylates.[1–3] In addition, rubbing the lens between the thumb and forefinger in a circular motion concentrates the abrasive action in the central portion of the lens, and minus power can be ground onto the lens over time.[1–4]

The most effective way to prevent these lens parameter changes is patient education on proper daily cleaning technique. The lens should be placed in the palm of the hand with a few drops of daily cleaner and rubbed in a back-and-forth, not circular, motion.[1–5] The patient should also concentrate on cleaning the lens edges. In doing so, the central portion will be cleaned too. To clean the concave surface, rub the lens in a radial fashion. Both surfaces should be cleaned for no more than 10–15 seconds each.[1–5]

Care system selection is important for RGP wearers. Less abrasive cleaners are recommended for softer, higher-Dk materials.[1–3] Boston Advance Comfort Formula and Alcon OptiSoak care systems use mildly abrasive daily cleaners that are less likely to cause parameter shifts. Lobob Optimum, Allergan Claris, and Allergan Wet-N-Soak Plus care systems use nonabrasive surfactant daily cleaners that are unlikely to cause lens changes. Lens material selection can further help prevent parameter changes. Material hardness indices such as Shore D and Rockwell can be helpful in differentiating materials.

Thoroughly questioning the patient about care systems and cleaning techniques, even experienced, long-term contact lens wearers, is important. This type of problem can be diagnosed and managed easily by first performing a comprehensive case history.

Clinical Pearls

- Vigorous daily cleaning with an abrasive cleaner can cause RGP parameter changes.
- A careful case history and good patient education can prevent recurrence of this problem.

References

1. Bennett ES, Henry VA. RGP lens power change with abrasive cleaner use. *Int Contact Lens Clin.* 1990;17(3):152–153.
2. Carrell BA, Bennett ES, Henry VA, Grohe RM. The effect of rigid gas-permeable lens cleaners on lens parameter stability. *J Am Optom Assoc.* 1992;63(3):193–198.

3. O'Donnell JJ. Patient-induced power changes in rigid gas-permeable contact lenses: A case report and literature review. *J Am Optom Assoc.* 1994;65(11):772–773.

4. Boltz KD. The overzealous contact lens cleaner. *Contact Lens Spectrum.* 1989;4(12):53–54.

5. Friedman DM. Too much lens cleaning can also be destructive. *Contact Lens Forum.* 1989;14(9):80.

Blurry Vision with New Rigid Gas-Permeable Contact Lenses

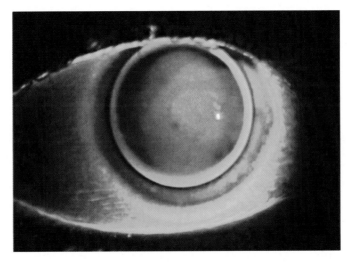

Figure 2-5

History

A 24-year-old Caucasian male presents for his 2-week follow-up on his new rigid gas-permeable (RGP) contact lenses (CL). He complains of blurry distance vision with the new lenses. He did not notice this blur with his old pair. He has worn RGP lenses for 6 years. The lenses are otherwise comfortable. His current average wear time is 13 hours per day. He is using Boston Advance Comfort Formula Care System. His ocular and medical histories are unremarkable. He takes no medications and is allergic to penicillin.

Symptoms

Distance blur with the new RGP lenses

Clinical Data

- Entering visual acuity with CL:
  OD 20/40
  OS 20/30
- Over-refraction:
  OD +0.75 –1.00 × 045, 20/20
  OS +0.75 –1.25 × 165, 20/20
- Over-keratometry:
  OD 38.25 / 39.00 @ 020
  OS 38.75 / 39.50 @ 063
- CL specifications:
  OD 7.80 / –1.25 / 9.0 / 0.11 / Polycon II
  OS 7.80 / –1.50 / 9.0 / 0.11 / Polycon II
- Keratometry (from previous visit):
  OD 42.25 / 44.25 @ 090
  OS 42.25 / 44.75 @ 090
- Subjective refraction (from previous visit):
  OD –0.25 –2.00 × 180, 20/25+
  OS –0.75 –2.50 × 180, 20/20–
- Gross external exam: Eyes appear white and quiet OU
- Biomicroscopy: All structures appear clear and healthy OU
- Fit assessment: OU—centered, blink movement 1 mm, apical clearance, mid-peripheral bearing, moderate peripheral clearance, moderate with-the-rule pattern (see Figure 2-5)

Develop your list of differential diagnoses. Then, based on the clinical data, determine your final diagnosis. Based on your diagnosis, develop your treatment plan.

Differential Diagnoses

- Lens switch
- RGP warpage
- RGP flexure
- Defective optics

Diagnosis

RGP flexure

Management

The patient was refitted with bitoric RGP contact lenses:

OD FluoroPerm 30 $\dfrac{7.94}{7.71} \Big/ \dfrac{\text{plano}}{-1.75}$ / 9.0 / 7.8 / 0.16

OS FluoroPerm 30 $\dfrac{7.94}{7.62} \Big/ \dfrac{-0.50}{-2.75}$ / 9.0 / 7.8 / 0.16

With the new lenses, the patient's visual acuity improved to OD 20/20– and OS 20/20 with over-refractions of OD plano –0.50 × 030 and OS plano sphere. The patient was pleased with his vision and continues to wear the lenses on a full-time schedule.

Discussion

The fitting of a moderately astigmatic cornea can sometimes result in flexure of a rigid contact lens. Flexure is caused by the mechanical bending of the lens due to hydrodynamic forces created by the lacrimal lens.[1] This is most significant when the lens centers on the cornea, creating a fulcrum-like effect over the corneal apex.[1–3] If flexible enough, the lens will bend instead of rocking on the cornea. The lacrimal lens is altered such that less of the corneal astigmatism is corrected. This usually results in residual astigmatism and a reduction in the patient's vision.

Factors that increase flexure include a central lens position,[1–5] moderate to high corneal toricity,[1–5] thin lens design,[6–8] large optic zone diameter,[9] and to some extent, eye lid tension.[1,4] Flexure is often unwanted because it can undercorrect the patient's astigmatism and result in blurry vision, as in this case. When a patient's astigmatism is all corneal, any reduction in astigmatic correction by the lacrimal lens results in poorer visual clarity. To improve the patient's vision, lens fit and design changes can be made to decrease flexure.

The simplest design change is to increase the center thickness of the lens by 0.03–0.04 mm.[4,6,7] This gives the lens added strength and rigidity and most likely will eliminate any significant lens flexure.

However, there are times when increasing lens thickness is undesirable. These may include a hyperopic prescription, history of corneal edema, or an inferior lens position. A thin lens design is preferable in each of these situations.

Other design changes that can be made include increasing lens diameter or using a higher modulus material. The larger lens will be more difficult to flex because of its greater size. The stiffer material will resist flexing even if you leave the lens design the same. The modulus can be determined by looking in a reference guide or calling your RGP laboratory. Dk value traditionally is thought to be predictive of lens hardness, but it is not a good predictor of lens flexure.[10,11]

One fit change that may help reduce flexure is a superior lid attachment.[4] By moving the lens center away from the "fulcrum" or apex of the cornea, flexure should decrease. This can be accomplished by flattening the posterior curves or increasing lens diameter. Minus carrier lenticular designs may also help, but take care not to decrease center thickness in the process.

Finally, a back surface toric or bitoric design can be used on corneas with at least 2.00 D of corneal cylinder. By more closely matching the corneal curvatures, the lens positions more centrally, has a smoother blink movement, and does not cause as much corneal molding.

Not all patients experience poor vision with lens flexure. In cases where the internal astigmatism is opposite to the corneal astigmatism, flexure is beneficial.[4] For example, a patient who has a with-the-rule cornea and refraction may have a keratometry reading of 43.00 / 46.00 @ 090 and a refraction of –3.00 –2.00 × 180. This patient has 1 diopter of against-the-rule astigmatism internally. If an RGP lens flexes by 1 diopter on this cornea, only 2 diopters are corrected by the lacrimal lens. Since the refraction has only 2 diopters of astigmatism, the patient will have no uncorrected astigmatism and will enjoy good acuity.

In cases where flexure may benefit the patient, lenses can be designed purposely to enhance flexure. By decreasing lens diameter and center thickness and by creating a central lens position with a steeper-than-K base curve, lens flexure will be maximized. Lower modulus RGP materials can be used as well. Flexure of up to one third to one half the corneal astigmatism can be generated by such a lens design.[1–4]

Clinical Pearls

- Flexure is increased with small, thin RGP designs and with a central lens position.

- Flexure is decreased by increasing center thickness, lens diameter, lens modulus, or by changing to a lid attachment fitting philosophy.
- Flexure may be beneficial when corneal and internal astigmatism are opposite.
- Lens flexure can be eliminated by refitting with a back toric design.

References

1. Corzine JC, Klein SA. Factors determining rigid contact lens flexure. *Optom Vis Sci.* 1997;74(8):639–645.
2. Herman JP. Flexure of rigid contact lenses on toric corneas as a function of base curve fitting relationship. *J Am Optom Assoc.* 1983;54(3):209–213.
3. Pole JJ. The effect of the base curve on the flexure of Polycon lenses. *Int Contact Lens Clin.* 1983;10(1):49–52.
4. Salmon TO. Beneficial flexure—using thin RGPs to correct residual astigmatism. *Contact Lens Spectrum.* 1992;7(8):39–42.
5. Harris MG. Contact lens flexure and residual astigmatism on toric corneas. *J Am Optom Assoc.* 1970;41(3):247–248.
6. Harris MG, Kadoya J, Nomura J, et al. Flexure and residual astigmatism with Polycon and polymethyl methacrylate lenses on toric corneas. *Am J Optom Physiol Opt.* 1982;59(3):263–266.
7. Harris MG, Chu CS. The effect of contact lens thickness and corneal toricity on flexure and residual astigmatism. *Am J Optom Arch Am Acad Optom.* 1972;49(4):304–307.
8. Harris MG, Appelquist TD. The effect of contact lens diameter and power on flexure and residual astigmatism. *Am J Optom Physiol Opt.* 1974;51(4):266–270.
9. Brown S, Baldwin M, Pole J. Effect of the optic zone diameter on lens flexure and residual astigmatism. *Int Contact Lens Clin.* 1984;11(12):759–763.
10. Sorbara L, Fonn D, MacNeill K. Effect of rigid gas-permeable lens flexure on vision. *Optom Vis Sci.* 1992;69(12):953–958.
11. Lin MC, Snyder C. Flexure and residual astigmatism with RGP lenses of low, medium, and high oxygen permeability. *Int Contact Lens Clin.* 1999;26(1):5–8.

CASE 2-6

Double Vision with Soft Toric Lenses

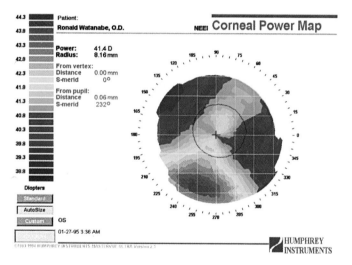

Figure 2-6

History

A 30-year-old Caucasian male presents for his 2-week progress evaluation for new soft toric contact lenses (CL). He is a previous soft toric lens wearer but presented at the last visit for a refit due to poor vision. At this visit, he complains of double images in both eyes that began 3 days after picking up his new lenses. The diplopia persists when he removes his lenses and wears his glasses. He has been wearing the lenses 10 hours per day with good comfort. He uses AOSept care system daily. He denies any ocular or medical history problems. He takes no medications and has no allergies.

Symptoms

Vertical monocular diplopia OU with contact lenses and glasses

Clinical Data

- Visual acuity with CL:
  OD 20/20
  OS 20/20
  Distinct ghost images OU
- CL specifications: Hydrasoft Toric DW,
  OD 8.9 / 15.0 / –2.25 –2.50 × 050
  OS 8.9 / 15.0 / –2.50 –2.50 × 165
- Pupils: PERRL – APD
- Over-refraction:
  OD Plano sphere, 20/20, ghost image still present
  OS +0.25 –0.50 × 115, 20/20, ghost image still present
- Fit assessment: OU centered with full coverage, 0.75 mm movement on blink, no rotation
- Biomicroscopy: OU all structures appear clear and healthy
- Corneal topography: OU inferior steep zone with superior flattening (see Figure 2-6)
- Keratometry:
  OD 40.00 / 42.75 @ 125, trace distortion
  OS 40.75 / 42.62 @ 070, trace distortion
- Subjective refraction:
  OD –2.50 –2.50 × 050, 20/20, ghost image still present
  OS –2.75 –2.00 × 150, 20/20, ghost image still present

Develop your list of differential diagnoses. Then, based on the clinical data, determine your final diagnosis. Based on your diagnosis, develop your treatment plan.

Differential Diagnoses

- Keratoconus
- Corneal warpage

Diagnosis

Corneal warpage

Management

Contact lens wear was discontinued. The patient's corneal topography and subjective refraction were monitored weekly. After 3 weeks, the double images disappeared and topography normalized. The patient was then refitted with aspheric rigid gas-permeable (RGP) contact lenses.

Boston Envision
OD 8.30 / –3.00 / 9.6
OS 8.20 / –3.25 / 9.6

With the new lenses, the patient noted blurry vision. Over-refraction and over-keratometry indicated that the RGP lenses were flexing on the eye. Bitoric RGP lenses were ordered and the patient was able to successfully adapt and wear them with good vision and comfort:

OD FluoroPerm 30 $\dfrac{8.18 / - 4.00}{8.60 / - 1.75}$ / 9.5 / 8.0

OS FluoroPerm 30 $\dfrac{8.10 / - 4.25}{8.38 / - 2.25}$ / 9.5 / 8.0

Discussion

Corneal warpage from contact lens wear is usually associated with rigid contact lenses. In most cases, a decentered lens position causes the cornea to be shifted such that the area under the lens flattens while the remainder of the cornea steepens. A superior lens position causes an inferior shift of the cornea, resulting in a topography similar to that of keratoconus. This is sometimes referred to as *pseudokeratoconus*.[1-4]

Although corneal warpage is not commonly associated with soft lenses, it can occur. Soft lens corneal warpage usually results from chronic wear of low Dk or thick-design lenses, often worn on an extended wear basis. However, thick soft toric lenses have also been associated with corneal warpage.[1,2] Because of the thickness of the lens, it can have significant effects on corneal shape. In addition, the lower Dk/L of these lenses, especially inferiorly, causes increased corneal hypoxia and edema, softening the cornea and predisposing it to mechanical shape changes,[1-3] which can occur quite rapidly, as in this case. The resulting corneal distortion causes blurry vision, ghost images, and in severe cases, diplopia.[1-3] This patient reported diplopia but, in fact, his symptoms were more consistent with distinct ghost images.

Resolution of the problem is simple once the diagnosis is made. But first, it must be differentiated from keratoconus and other corneal degenerative conditions that may cause a similar change in corneal topography.[1-4] Although similar to keratoconus, contact lens–induced corneal warpage is different in several ways. First, its time course follows initiation of contact lens wear, while keratoconus may or may not be associated with contact lens wear. Second, the overall corneal curvature does not change; instead, one portion steepens while another flattens by approximately the same amount. In keratoconus, the inferior cornea thins and steepens while the remainder of the cornea remains relatively normal. Third, there are no visible corneal signs in corneal warpage, while keratoconus may be characterized by findings such as Vogt's striae, Fleischer ring, and scarring. Finally, corneal warpage will resolve, while keratoconus tends to progress, even in the absence of a contact lens.

When refitting lenses on a patient with corneal warpage, consider the cause of the condition and prevention of future changes. Because this patient wears a thick, large-diameter soft toric lens, refitting to a similar design should be avoided. A smaller, thinner design with less prism ballast or a thin-zone design with no prism ballast can be fit. We decided to fit the patient with a well-centered aspheric RGP contact lens. Although RGPs may also cause warpage, a centrally fitting lens causes no asymmetric corneal shift, which would lead to ghost images and diplopia. Expected changes would include spon change of the cornea. Neither change would induce ghosting while the lenses were worn, although a spectacle prescription change would likely be needed. In this case, the aspheric design failed as well, due to high corneal astigmatism and lens flexure. The patient was then refit into a bitoric design with good success.

Clinical Pearls

- Soft lenses can induce corneal warpage.
- Contact lens warpage must be differentiated from corneal degenerations, such as keratoconus.
- Serial corneal topography is important in the management of corneal warpage.

References

1. Hagan S, Kirks M, Johnson J. Corneal warpage (pseudokeratoconus) and soft toric contact lenses: A case report. *Int Contact Lens Clin.* 1998;25(4):114–116.

2. Lebow KA, Grohe RM. Differentiating contact lens–induced warpage from true keratoconus using corneal topography. *CLAO J.* 1999;25(2):114–122.
3. Shovlin JP, DePaolis MD, Kame RT. Contact lens–induced corneal warpage syndrome vs. keratoconus. *Contact Lens Forum.* 1986;11(8):32–36.
4. Eghbali F. Keratoconus suspect or pseudokeratoconus? *Contact Lens Spectrum.* 1997;12(12):30–32.

Cloudy Vision

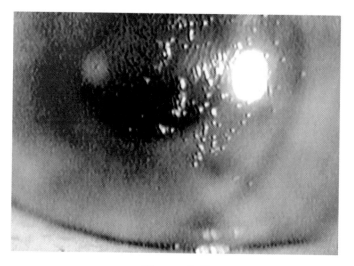

Figure 2-7

History

A 45-year-old Caucasian female presents with complaints of cloudy vision with her rigid gas-permeable (RGP) contact lenses (CL). Her current lenses are 2 years old. She has noticed a gradual clouding of her vision but has no other complaints. The lenses are comfortable, and she denies redness, irritation, or pain. She uses the Boston Simplicity care system and wears her lenses 16 hours per day. Her ocular and medical histories are unremarkable. She takes no medications and has no allergies.

Symptoms

Cloudy vision with RGP lenses

Clinical Data

- Entering visual acuity with CL:
  OD 20/30
  OS 20/40
- Over-refraction:
  OD Plano –0.50 × 170, 20/30
  OS Plano sphere, 20/40
- CL Specifications:
  OD 7.70 / –4.50 / 9.6 / Boston 7 Envision
  OS 7.70 / –5.75 / 9.6 / Boston 7 Envision
- Keratometry:
  OD 44.25 / 45.25 @ 080
  OS 44.50 / 45.00 @ 100
- Subjective refraction:
  OD –5.00 –0.75 × 165, 20/20
  OS –6.50 –0.50 × 010, 20/20
- Gross external exam: Eyes appear white and quiet OU
- Biomicroscopy: Moderate meibomian gland dysfunction, thick eyeliner along lid margins, all other structures appear clear and healthy OU
- Fit assessment: OU Superior central, blink movement 2 mm, apical touch, mid-peripheral clearance, moderate peripheral clearance, greasy surface deposits (see Figure 2-7)

Develop your list of differential diagnoses. Then, based on the clinical data, determine your final diagnosis. Based on your diagnosis, develop your treatment plan.

Differential Diagnoses

- Protein deposit
- Surface contamination
- Meibomian gland dysfunction
- Corneal edema
- Posterior segment complication

Diagnosis

Surface contamination with makeup and hair spray

Management

New lenses in a lower Dk fluorosilicone acrylate material (Boston ES) were ordered. The patient's care system was changed to the Boston Advance Comfort Formula with weekly liquid enzyme. Nightly lid hygiene with warm compresses, lid massage, and lid scrubs was prescribed. She was advised to modify her makeup application habits so as not to apply anything behind the lash line and to close her eyes when applying hair spray. She now enjoys clear vision with her lenses.

Discussion

Fluorosilicone acrylate materials have been of great benefit to rigid contact lens wearers. They have greater oxygen permeability and protein resistance than silicone acrylate materials. However, the fluorine makes these materials more lipophilic, which often causes oily, greasy deposits to build up on the lens surface.[1] This is exacerbated by patients who use lotions and makeup around the eyes. It is further aggravated by abnormal tears, specifically, abnormal meibomian gland secretions and dry eye. The result is a lens surface layered with a greasy film that is hydrophobic. The lens does not wet properly, resulting in cloudy, blurry vision.[2]

An in-depth case history is the first step in determining the source of the contamination. The patient should be questioned about her makeup application habits, the type of makeup and lotions or hair sprays used, and any other solutions or chemicals applied to or near the eyelids. In addition, a description of the patient's daily routine of facial hygiene and contact lens application and removal should be obtained. Is the patient wearing her lenses when makeup is applied, or does she apply the lenses after her makeup? Is she wearing her lenses while using hair spray? Does she use hand lotion prior to lens handling? If so, these behaviors should be changed. Finally, does the patient clean her eyelids at night? If her makeup is not removed, it is more likely to contaminate her lenses the next day.[2,3]

Management is based on the clinical findings. A careful assessment of the lid margins and tear film structure and function should be made. Makeup applied inside the lash line can spill into the tear prism and contaminate the lens. Clogged or inflamed meibomian glands signify poor or abnormal production of the tear film's lipid layer. Express the glands to examine the quality of the meibum. If it is anything other than clear, warm compresses, lid massage, and lid scrubs should be prescribed. Examine tear breakup time, use Schirmer's or phenol red-thread test, and look for corneal and conjunctival staining with fluorescein and lissamine green dyes to determine if the patient has dry eyes. Dry eye is more likely to cause deposits to form on the lens surface. Finally, assess the patient's blink habits. If the blinks are infrequent or incomplete, the lens surface may be drying out and increasing the likelihood of deposit formation.

The next component in effective management is the care system. A multipurpose system like Simplicity is not as effective as a two-step system in removing surface deposits like protein and lipids. Changing to a care system with a separate daily cleaner allows the patient to better clean his or her lenses. Addition of a liquid enzyme also may help, by keeping lipophilic protein from coating the lens.

Finally, lens material selection should be considered. A high-Dk fluorosilicone acrylate material, like Boston 7, may not be the best choice for a person with lipid deposition problems. Consider a lipophilic material or even a silicone acrylate to minimize lipid deposition.

Clinical Pearls

- Makeup, lotions, and hair spray may create a greasy film that causes cloudy vision.
- Multipurpose solutions may not be effective enough to prevent buildup of makeup.
- Effective management of lipid buildup may include extensive patient education, care system modification, and lens material selection.

References

1. Bontempo AR, Rapp J. Lipid deposits on hydrophilic and rigid gas-permeable contact lenses. *CLAO J.* 1994;20(4):242–245.
2. Tlachac CA. Cosmetics and contact lenses. *Optom Clin.* 1994;4(1):35–45.
3. Baldwin JS. Cosmetics: Too long concealed as culprit in eye problems. *Contact Lens Forum.* 1986;11(6):38–41.

CASE 2-8

Foggy Vision

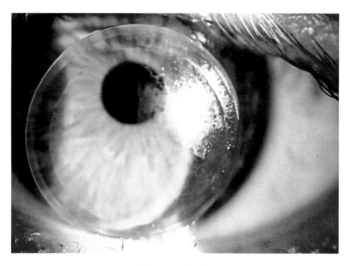

Figure 2-8

History

A 54-year-old Caucasian male presents for a 6-month progress evaluation on his rigid gas-permeable (RGP) contact lenses (CL). He states that the lenses are comfortable but, occasionally, the lenses fog up or cloud over. He cleans the lenses vigorously every night with Boston Advance Daily Cleaner, but the lenses still seem to cloud. His vision is clear when the lenses are not foggy. These problems began about 2 weeks prior to his visit. He is in good general health, takes no medications, and has no allergies.

Symptoms

Foggy, cloudy vision with RGP contact lenses

Clinical Data

- Entering visual acuity with CL:
  OD 20/40
  OS 20/25
- Over-refraction:
  OD +0.25 –0.25 × 090, 20/40
  OS Plano –0.50 × 180, 20/20–
- CL specifications: OU 7.90 / –3.50 / 9.5 / 8.0 / Boston ES
- Keratometry:
  OD 43.50 / 43.75 @ 090
  OS 43.00 sphere
- Subjective refraction:
  OD –4.50 sphere, 20/20
  OS –4.00 –0.50 × 090, 20/20
- Gross external exam: Eyes appear white and quiet OU
- Biomicroscopy: Grade 3 meibomian gland dysfunction OU, grade 2 blepharitis OU, grade 1 lid erythema along lid margins; all other structures appear clear and healthy OU
- Fit assessment: OU superior central lid attachment, blink movement 2 mm, apical alignment, mid-peripheral alignment, moderate peripheral clearance, surface nonwetting (see Figure 2-8)

Develop your list of differential diagnoses. Then, based on the clinical data, determine your final diagnosis. Based on your diagnosis, develop your treatment plan.

Differential Diagnoses

- Protein deposit
- Surface contamination
- Meibomian gland dysfunction
- Corneal edema

Diagnosis

RGP surface contamination and nonwetting due to meibomitis

Management

The patient's lenses were cleaned with an alcohol-based cleaner to remove surface deposits. His care system was changed to Lobob

Optimum with Supraclens liquid enzyme twice a week. He was also given a lid hygiene regimen and more extensive education on the reasons for his cloudy vision. Over the next several months, a significant improvement in lid health and vision was noted. However, the patient still has signs of meibomitis and blepharitis, which he continues to work on.

Discussion

Surface nonwetting is a common problem with modern fluorosilicone acrylate RGP materials.[1,2] The lens surface is easily contaminated by oils, lipids, and other greasy substances like makeup, lotions, and meibomian gland oils. When a patient has moderate to severe meibomian gland dysfunction, excessive meibum can be secreted, which can accumulate on the lens surface. The resulting lens surface is irregular and hydrophobic, and the tear film cannot spread evenly across it. In addition, tear film evaporation is increased.[3] As a result, light cannot refract properly through the lens, resulting in cloudy or foggy vision[4-6] and, in some cases, lens intolerance.[7] This reduced vision cannot be corrected by over-refraction. The solution is to clean the lens and prevent its recontamination.

The first consideration is the patient's eyelid condition. This patient has moderate to severe meibomian gland dysfunction and blepharitis. The traditional therapies of hot compresses, lid scrubs, and lid massage help reduce the severity of the conditions. However, severe cases of meibomitis may require an oral antibiotic, such as doxycycline or minocycline, to improve the meibomian secretions. Topical antibiotic ointments, such as bacitracin or erythromycin, may help resolve a stubborn blepharitis, while an antibiotic-steroid combination ointment, such as Tobradex, may be needed in a severely inflamed and painful blepharitis.[8] Once the condition has been controlled, the patient must be advised that continued lid hygiene is crucial in maintaining healthy eyelid margins and clean contact lens surfaces.[7,8] A maintenance regimen of at least two or three times per week is necessary to keep the lids healthy. Cessation of lid hygiene almost always results in a return of symptoms.

The second course of action is to clean the contact lens and provide the patient with an optimal cleaning regimen for long-term use. Alcohol-based cleaners, such as the Boston Laboratory Lens Cleaner and MiraFlow Extra Strength Daily Cleaner, are very effective in removing oily, greasy films and deposits from the RGP surface. However, they are not recommended for daily use because the lens materials cannot withstand frequent use of the harsh solvents. An in-office lens cleaning routine should include vigorous cleaning with an alcohol-based cleaner, a second cleaning with an RGP daily cleaner, and a soak in a conditioning or wetting solution. Once the lens surface is clean and wet, the patient will notice vastly improved vision.

The patient should also be given a new cleaning regimen for everyday use. Because the Boston care system seems not to have been effective by itself, one possible recommendation is to supplement it with a periodic cleaning with an alcohol-based cleaner, even though these cleaners are not recommended for dispensing to the patient. This will allow the patient to do the equivalent of your in-office cleaning at home. This recommendation should be accompanied by a warning that the lens may not last as long and therefore require more frequent replacement. Another recommendation is to supplement the care system with a daily or weekly enzymatic cleaning. While this does not directly affect deposition of the lipid on the lens surface, it may be of benefit by maintaining a protein-free lens surface. A clean lens surface is less likely to allow other deposits (and microorganisms) to collect on the lens, and even though RGP lenses do not readily attract protein deposits, higher-Dk materials with higher silicone content may benefit from enzyme cleaner usage. Finally, a change to a different system can be recommended. Benzyl alcohol-based systems, such as Lobob Optimum and Allergan Claris, work with surfactants to clean the lens surface of lipoidal deposits. When combined with an enzymatic cleaner, they can be very effective against lipid deposits.

The final consideration in this case is the lens material. Although Boston ES is an excellent material with many good characteristics, it can have wetting problems in patients with marginal tear qualities. A change to a material with a more favorable wetting angle should be considered. In this case, the addition of the lid hygiene regimen and the change in contact lens care regimen were effective in eliminating the patient's symptoms. However, if the patient had continued to experience foggy vision, a material change would have been made. In contrast, a change in lens material without the other two changes would not have solved the patient's problem, because it would not have addressed the symptom's etiology, which was the poor condition of the lids.

Clinical Pearls

- Cloudy or foggy vision with RGP contact lenses often is due to surface nonwetting caused by contaminants.

- The etiology of the surface contamination must be addressed to effectively eliminate the patient's symptoms.
- Long-term lid hygiene is crucial in treating meibomitis and blepharitis.
- Care systems and lens materials play an important role in reducing surface nonwetting.

References

1. Bontempo AR, Rapp J. Protein-lipid interaction on the surface of a rigid gas-permeable contact lens in vitro. *Curr Eye Res.* 1997;16(12):1258–1262.
2. Bontempo AR, Rapp J. Lipid deposits on hydrophilic and rigid gas-permeable contact lenses. *CLAO J.* 1994;20(4):242–245.
3. Mathers WD. Ocular evaporation in meibomian gland dysfunction and dry eye. *Ophthalmol.* 1993;100(3):347–351.
4. Korb D, Henriquez A. Meibomian gland dysfunction and contact lens intolerance. *J Am Optom Assoc.* 1980;51(3):243–251.
5. Grohe RM, Caroline PJ. RGP non-wetting lens syndrome. *Contact Lens Spectrum.* 1989;4(3):32.
6. Snyder C. Preocular tear film anomalies and lens-related dryness. In: Silbert JA (ed). *Anterior Segment Complications of Contact Lens Wear*, 2nd ed. Boston: Butterworth–Heinemann, 2000:3–21.
7. Paugh JR, Knapp LL, Martinson JR, Hom MM. Meibomian therapy in problematic contact lens wear. *Optom Vis Sci.* 1990; 67(11):803–806.
8. Driver PJ, Lemp MA. Meibomian gland dysfunction. *Surv Ophthalmol.* 1996;40(5):343–367.

Blurry Near Vision

Neil A. Pence

History

Patient RT is a school administrator with a history of 19 years of daily wear of soft contact lenses (CL) without complication. She is in general good health, and her ocular health history is normal and unremarkable. RT reported, at age 44, wearing single-vision soft contact lenses. She was largely asymptomatic, with some mild reading problems in poor light or at the end of a very long day. Entering distance acuities with contact lenses were

OD 20/20 with a −3.50 CL; over-refraction: −0.25 sphere, 20/15
OS 20/20+ with a −3.25 CL; over-refraction: −0.25 sphere, 20/15

Subjective refraction was OD −3.75 sphere, 20/15, and OS −3.50 sphere, 20/15, with a near BVA with a +0.50 add.

RT was given the option of slightly improving her distance vision with a lens power change, at the expense of her near comfort. She chose, however, to continue in her current contact lens powers, since she was basically happy with her vision and was experiencing few difficulties.

RT returned 14 months later at age 45. She noted increased reading difficulty, more fatigue with near work, and inability to read very small print.

Symptoms

RT has difficulty at near with her current soft contact lenses

Clinical Data

- Entering visual acuity with contact lenses:
  OD 20/20 at distance; 20/40 at near
  OS 20/20 at distance; 20/40 at near
- Over-refraction:
  OD –0.25 at distance; +0.75 at near
  OS –0.25 at distance; +0.75 at near
- Subjective refraction:
  OD –3.75 –0.25 × 80, 20/15
  OS –3.50 sphere, 20/15
  +1.00 add

Diagnosis

Emerging presbyopia

Management

Three contact lens options were discussed with RT:

1. Single-vision contact lenses (increased –0.25 OU) and reading glasses
2. Monovision with single-vision contact lenses
3. Bifocal contact lenses

It was decided to first evaluate the patient's initial reaction to monovision. Determining that RT was both sighting and focusing dominant with her right eye made it a good choice to start with for distance vision. Sighting dominance was determined with the "hole-in-the-hand test" (overlap the two hands to form a small circle above the thumbs, push the hands out to arm's length, raise them up to view the examiner's nose through the circle; then the examiner can see which eye is looking through the hole—that is the dominant sighting eye). Focusing dominance was determined by the "+1.50 lens test" (view a distance chart with both eyes open and best corrected; alternately, place a +1.50 trial lens in front of each eye and ask on which side vision is more affected by the lens—that eye is the dominant eye with regard to focusing).

RT was given contact lenses as follows:

OD –3.75, 20/15 distance acuity
OS –2.50, 20/20 near acuity

At a 1-week follow-up visit, RT reported good adaptation to and satisfaction with monovision. Visual acuities are

OD 20/15 at distance; over-refraction: plano sphere, 20/15
OS 20/20– at near; over-refraction: +0.25 sphere, 20/20

With both eyes open and lenses on, RT reports better vision on a near card with a +0.25 lens held in front of the left eye. RT still exhibits a good range at near as well. When viewing the distance chart, RT reports that distance vision also is improved when the +0.25 lens is in front of the left eye (the near eye). RT is dispensed a 6-month supply of contact lenses with the following lens powers: OD –3.75, OS –2.25. At both 1-month and 6-month visits, RT reports doing fine with her monovision contact lens system and experiences no particular problems or difficulties.

Discussion

Several points in the case of RT may be informative. First, she represents one of the approaches that may be employed for the early or emerging presbyope. At age 44, she was very slightly undercorrected for distance vision, which gave her a small benefit with regard to near. When this is the case, it often is beneficial to leave the patient underminused until he or she becomes more symptomatic for near problems. This is especially true when the patient has no distance complaints, as in this case. It might be suggested that monovision should have been tried at age 44, but since all forms of presbyopic contact lens correction represent some form of compromise, clinical experience suggests that patients accept this compromise best if they know they have to. RT had relatively few complaints, and until she was bothered more significantly with her near vision, she would be less likely to accept other forms of correction.

Similarly, if RT had been fully corrected for distance at age 44 and cutting her distance by 0.25 D had been tried, she would have been aware of giving up some distance acuity. While on occasion, this may be successful, it usually is more difficult; and if a compromise is to be given, it might be best to begin the patient in monovision at that point.

The second interesting aspect of this case involves the seemingly paradoxical situation of adding more plus to the near eye, making it obviously less well focused for distance viewing, and having the patient report that it improves their distance vision. While unexpected, it turns out that this finding is not rare or unusual when dealing with monovision fits, especially when relatively low adds are being corrected.

One theory regarding monovision fits is that it is best to minimize the difference between the two eyes. This makes it more similar to the normal binocular state and also seems to be less objectionable to some practitioners. Because the distance acuity is going to be compromised roughly 7 to 10% by having only one eye focused for distance, it is generally accepted that the full correction must be given to the distance eye. Therefore, to minimize the difference between the two eyes, a slightly weaker add has to be given the near eye.[1]

While this may sound and "feel" good, RT is a good example of a monovision patient doing better when we make the two eyes a little more different, not less different. When the difference is relatively small (i.e., for lower additions or new presbyopes), monovision works best when the brain can clearly discern to which eye it is supposed to direct its concentration. If the disparity is less, it is more difficult for the brain to pick out one eye's focus. Increasing the add helps the visual system to more easily determine which eye is to be paid more attention for a given distance. Clinical experience suggests that this is true for adds of +1.50 D or less. Some of the explanation for this may relate to the fact that binocular summation is still relatively good up to about a +1.75 D add.[2] Therefore, binocular summation may be too strong to allow good monovision adaptation to occur in lower addition powers. By making the two eyes more clearly different, patients seem to better "choose" the eye that is to get more attention in terms of focus.

When fitting monovision for patients with add powers in the +0.75 to +1.25 D range, like this patient, it has been suggested that increasing the monovision add power first given may aid adaptation.[3] At the very least, clinicians should not be surprised when the apparent paradox represented here occurs. When dealing with first-time monovision fits of later presbyopes (+2.00 D add or higher), there may be some advantage in lessening the amount of disparity given. Anecdotal clinical findings suggest slightly less satisfaction with monovision when higher add powers are needed, presumably due to the significant drop-off of binocular summation after a +1.75 D add. Therefore, it is reasonable to cut the add power given for first-time monovision trials in these more mature presbyopes. These patients also are more likely to be candidates for various forms of modified monovision as well.

Clinical Pearls

- Underminusing early presbyopes to enhance near vision is more successful if they already are accustomed to being undercorrected.

- Some early monovision patients report improvement in their distance vision when increasing the plus in their near eye; the larger difference between eyes allows them to more easily determine the proper eye to use at each distance.
- The reading power should be cut slightly in presbyopes requiring higher add powers.

References

1. Snyder C. Monovision: A clinical view. *Contact Lens Spectrum.*1989;4(4):30.
2. Loshin DS, Loshin MS, Comer G. Binocular summation with monovision contact lens correction for presbyopia. *Int Contact Lens Clin.* 1982;9(3):161–165.
3. Pence NA. Strategies for success with presbyopes. *Contact Lens Spectrum.*1994;9(5):30, 39.

More Problems with Near Vision

History

Patient ML, a 45-year-old female, presents for her annual eye examination with complaints of poor near vision with her current contact lenses (CL). She currently wears soft lenses on a daily basis. She says that she is having problems focusing at work, where she does paperwork and computer data entry. The lenses are comfortable, and she can wear them 14 hours per day. She uses OptiFree Express to clean and disinfect the lenses. She denies any ocular problems. Her ocular history is unremarkable. She has hypothyroidism, for which she takes Synthroid. She has no allergies.

Symptoms

Poor near vision with her current soft contact lenses

Clinical Data

- Entering visual acuity at distance with CL:
  OD 20/20
  OS 20/20
- Entering visual acuity at near with CL:
  OD 20/50
  OS 20/50
- Contact lens parameters:
  OD Focus Monthly 8.6 / 14.0 / –4.25
  OS Focus Monthly 8.6 / 14.0 / –3.75
- Over-refraction at distance:
  OD Plano sphere, 20/20
  OS +0.25 –0.50 × 090, 20/20

- Over-refraction at near:
  OD +1.25 sphere, 20/20
  OS +1.50 –0.50 × 090, 20/20
- Fit assessment: OU centered, 0.5 mm movement on blink, clear lens surfaces
- Keratometry
  OD 43.50 / 44.25 @ 090
  OS 43.75 / 44.00 @ 090
- Subjective refraction:
  OD –4.50 sphere, 20/20
  OS –3.50 –0.50 × 090, 20/20
  +1.50 add
- External exam: All structures appear white and quiet OU
- Biomicroscopy: All structures appear white and quiet OU

Diagnosis

Presbyopia

Management

Because of the patient's difficulty with her near vision on the job, she was refit with a multifocal soft contact lens OS only. Her left eye was found to be nondominant. This modified monovision system allowed her to maintain her binocularity at distance while improving near acuity. The new lens for OS was Focus Progressive 8.6 / 14.0 / –3.00.

The patient's visual acuity with this new lens was 20/25– at distance and 20/25 at near. Binocularly, the patient was 20/20 at distance and 20/25 at near. The patient wore this new left lens with her existing right lens and was scheduled for a follow-up visit. At this visit, she reported that she would like a little clearer near vision. Over-refraction with +0.25 over the OS gave her 20/30 at distance and 20/20 at near, and binocularly she attained 20/20 at distance and near.

Discussion

Early presbyopes have several options for contact lens correction, including monovision, multifocal contact lenses, and reading glasses. Monovision provides improved near acuity but may decrease distance acuity, and adaptation is sometimes difficult,[1] especially for those requiring high add powers.[2,3] In addition, the ethical questions surrounding the fitting of monovision for moderate to high presbyopia have not yet been resolved.[4] Multifocal lenses improve near vision binocularly but tend to decrease distance vision, especially with soft lens designs. Low to moderate presbyopes may be well served by fitting them with a single-vision lens for distance in one eye and a multifocal lens in the other.[5] This modified monovision system benefits the patient by maintaining most of the patient's binocularity at distance while providing plus for near in the nondominant eye. In addition, it is a good option for patients who do not like the idea of blurring one eye with monovision.

The fitting of modified monovision can take several forms, but one common method is to leave the patient in a single-vision distance lens on the dominant eye while fitting the nondominant eye with a multifocal lens.[5] An aspheric lens design is selected to provide both near and intermediate powers. The fitting process should be prefaced by a discussion of what the patient should expect to see. In most cases, a compromise in distance vision must be tolerated. This is generally less blurred than monovision but noticeably different from single-vision distance-only lenses. If the patient is willing to proceed, an appropriate lens design and power should be selected and placed on the eye. After 15–20 minutes of settling time, if the patient appears to be doing well at both distance and near, he or she should be scheduled for a follow-up visit. At the follow-up visit, the visual assessment includes binocular visual acuity at distance and near and an over-refraction. The over-refraction is performed with room lights on and both eyes open. If the lens power is selected properly, the patient should be no more than ±0.50 D away from the final power. Successful patients report that, although their vision is not perfect, they can see well enough to perform almost all their visual tasks. In this case, the patient could read her paperwork and focus well on the computer screen. She had difficulty with fine print, but she rarely performed this type of visual task. She was advised to have some low plus readers made for those instances when she needed to see fine detail.

Fitting one eye with a multifocal lens often provides an easier transition for early presbyopes than binocular fitting of multifocal lenses. Because their near add requirements still are relatively low, they can see well with only one eye corrected for near. As they get older and their add requirements increase, they may require binocular multifocal fitting to attain sufficient near point clarity. By starting with one multifocal lens, it is an easier transition to fit both eyes.

Clinical Pearls

- Modified monovision is an effective contact lens option for early presbyopes.
- In modified monovision, a multifocal lens is fit on the nondominant eye.
- Patients fit with modified monovision must be given proper visual expectations for multifocal lenses.

References

1. Collins M, Bruce A, Thompson B. Adaptation to monovision. *Int Contact Lens Clin.* 1994;21(6):218–223.
2. Collins MJ, Bruce AS. Factors influencing performance with monovision. *J Brit Contact Lens Assoc.* 1994;17(3):83–89.
3. Back A. Factors influencing success and failure in monovision. *Int Contact Lens Clin.* 1995;22(4):165–172.
4. Koetting RA. The safety of monovision. *Prac Optom.* 1999;10(1):10–13.
5. Fisher K. Presbyopic visual performance with modified monovision using multifocal soft contact lenses. *Int Contact Lens Clin.* 1997;24(3):91–99.

PART 3

Fit-Induced Complications

CASE 3-1

Soft Lens Red Eye

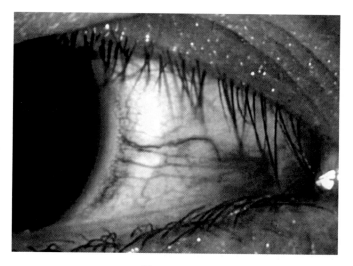

Figure 3-1

History

Patient MD is a 25-year-old Asian male. He presents for the first time with complaints of redness and irritation while wearing his soft contact lenses (CL). He reports that the irritation worsens later in the day and with each additional day of wear. He also notes that he has difficulty removing the lenses at the end of his wearing time. He has been wearing soft contact lenses for 8 years on an extended-wear schedule. His average wearing time is 7 consecutive days, and his current wearing time is 3 days. At the end of the week, he cleans and disinfects his lenses with AOSept and uses an enzymatic cleaner. He replaces his lenses every 3 months, and his current lenses are 2 months old. His ocular and medical histories are otherwise unremarkable. He takes no medications and has no allergies.

Symptoms

Redness and irritation after several hours of wear

Clinical Findings

- Visual acuity with contact lenses:
  OD 20/20
  OS 20/20
- Contact lens parameters:
  OD: Focus / 8.6 / –5.00 / 14.0
  OS: Focus / 8.6 / –4.00 / 14.0
- Contact lens fit assessment: Central position, no movement on blink, no lag movement, minimal movement on push-up test, mild surface deposition OU
- Keratometry (after CL removal):
  OD 42.75 / 43.50 @ 090
  OS 42.50 / 43.00 @ 080
- Subjective refraction without CL:
  OD –5.00 –1.00 × 180, 20/20
  OS –4.25 –0.25 × 170, 20/20
- Biomicroscopy: Grade 2 diffuse bulbar injection, trace limbal corneal staining superiorly, grade 1 vascularization 360° OU (see Figure 3-1)

Based on the clinical data, develop your list of differential diagnoses. Then, determine your final diagnosis and develop your treatment plan.

Differential Diagnoses

- Tight-fitting soft lens
- Soft lens desiccation
- Contact lens acute red eye
- Soft-lens-associated chronic hypoxia
- Giant papillary conjunctivitis
- Superior limbic keratoconjunctivitis
- Solution-preservative sensitivity

Diagnosis

Tight-fitting soft contact lens exacerbated by extended wear

Management

Because the patient had not yet developed a "severe" complication, a conservative management approach was taken. First, the patient was instructed to discontinue lens wear for 7 days or until injection and staining resolve. He was prescribed artificial tears qid for 7 days. After resolution of the injection and staining, he was refitted with Focus lenses with an 8.9 mm base curve. His wear time was reduced to three consecutive nights maximum, and he was instructed to replace his lenses every month. He was seen for follow-up visits at 1 week and 1 month, then advised to return every 6 months thereafter to monitor lens fit and ocular health.

Discussion

Tight-fitting soft contact lenses can cause a myriad of ocular complications.[1,2] In many cases, the lenses may fit well initially, but over the course of several months, the contact lenses begin to adhere. This is accelerated by extended wear because the lenses dry out more than with overnight wear. In this case, the patient luckily has not yet manifested serious problems. However, the bulbar injection and superior corneal staining are signs that further problems are impending. Discontinuation of lens wear until the staining and injection resolve is the best first course of action. Artificial tears may help soothe the eyes and promote epithelial healing. The major issues in this case are the tight fit and the extended wear. The tight fit can be addressed by simply refitting to a flatter base curve. However, extended wear may be the greater issue in causing the lenses to tighten. Since the patient is not yet manifesting more serious and chronic complications such as microcysts, severe neovascularization and infiltrates, extended wear with a looser fitting lens may be acceptable. It would be advisable to instruct the patient to decrease the number of consecutive nights he wears his lenses and most desirable to have the patient change to a daily-wear schedule. In addition, more frequent lens replacement, such as 1 month as recommended by the manufacturer, would reduce the surface deposits that may be contributing to the patient's problems.

Giant papillary conjunctivitis is a possible cause of this patient's symptoms,[1,2] but lack of hyperemia and papillae on the upper palpebral conjunctiva help rule out this condition. Superior limbic keratoconjunctivitis also causes irritation and redness, although the redness is localized to the superior bulbar conjunctiva.[1,2] Solution preservative sensitivity also causes irritation and diffuse redness, although the patient will complain of stinging or burning soon after lens insertion, not later in the day. This can be ruled out by changing the care system and monitoring signs and symptoms. Finally, lens dryness can cause similar symptoms, but with the obvious tight lens fit, it can be ruled out as the primary cause of the patient's symptoms. However, it is likely to be a contributing factor.

Contact lens acute red eye (CLARE) is a unilateral soft lens complication characterized by severe pain, photophobia, tearing, and redness, usually on waking in the early morning.[1-3] Although epithelial staining sometimes is absent, subepithelial infiltrates usually are present. This inflammatory response is thought to be due to bacteria and their toxins being trapped behind a tightly fitting lens. Soft lens–associated chronic hypoxia (SLACH) is a syndrome in which loosely adherent corneal epithelium is removed along with the soft lens being removed.[4] The result is a poorly healing corneal abrasion due to long-term hypoxia caused by extended wear of low-Dk soft lenses.

As extensively documented, extended wear of soft contact lenses puts the patient at significantly higher risk of complications.[2] All potential complications of tight-fitting contact lenses are more likely to occur with extended wear. Because tight lenses may just be a portent of more severe problems, early detection and refitting are important, especially with extended-wear lenses.

Clinical Pearls

- A tight-fitting soft contact lens may result in symptoms of redness and irritation.
- Long-term complications due to tight-fitting soft lenses may include microcysts, neovascularization, and infiltrates.
- Extended wear exacerbates tight lens– and deposit-related complications.

References

1. Silbert JA. Inflammatory responses in contact lens wear. In: Silbert JA (ed). *Anterior Segment Complications of Contact Lens Wear*, 2nd ed. Boston: Butterworth–Heinemann, 2000:109–131.
2. Swarbrick HA, Holden BA. Complications of hydrogel extended-wear lenses. In: Silbert JA (ed). *Anterior Segment Complications of Contact Lens Wear*, 2nd ed. Boston: Butterworth–Heinemann, 2000:273–308.

3. Holden BA, LaHood D, Grant T, et al. Gram-negative bacteria can induce contact lens related acute red eye (CLARE) responses. *CLAO J*. 1996;22(1):47–52.
4. Wallace W. The SLACH syndrome. *Int Eyecare*. 1985;1(3):220.

Pain with Soft Lens Wear

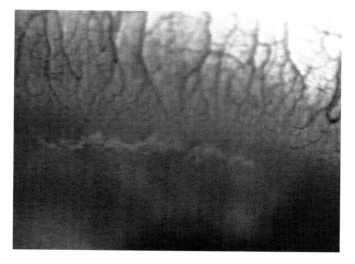

Figure 3-2

History

A 35-year-old Asian male presents with symptoms of moderate sharp pain in his right eye since the day before. He reports no blurry vision, no mucous discharge, no photophobia, and no visible redness. He was fit 10 days earlier with PureVision silicone hydrogel contact lenses (CL) to be worn on an extended-wear basis for 7 days/6 nights. On his 1 week progress evaluation, no problems were noted. After the progress evaluation, he removed his lenses, cleaned and disinfected them, and reinserted them the following morning. His current wearing time is 3 days. He previously had been a successful daily disposable soft lens wearer. His ocular and medical histories are unremarkable. He takes no medications and has an allergy to penicillin.

Symptoms

Moderate sharp pain for 2 days

Clinical Data

- Visual acuity with CL:
  OD 20/15
  OS 20/15
- CL specifications: OU PureVision / 8.6 / 14.0 / –3.75
- Pupils: PERRL-APD
- Over-refraction:
  OD Plano sphere, 20/15
  OS Plano sphere, 20/15
- Contact lens fit: OU centered, 0.5 mm movement on blink, good push-up movement
- Biomicroscopy:
  OD: Superior bulbar injection, linear corneal epithelial lesion parallel to the limbus that stains with fluorescein (see Figure 3-2)
  OS: All structures appear normal
- Keratometry (from previous visit):
  OD 41.50 / 42.25 @ 090
  OS 41.75 / 42.00 @ 090
- Subjective refraction (from previous visit):
  OD –4.00 –0.50 × 180, 20/15
  OS –3.75 –0.50 × 180, 20.15

Based on the clinical data, develop your list of differential diagnoses. Then, determine your final diagnosis and develop your treatment plan.

Differential Diagnoses

- Superior limbic keratoconjunctivitis
- Superior epithelial arcuate lesion
- Contact lens acute red eye
- Soft-lens-associated chronic hypoxia
- Giant papillary conjunctivitis
- Solution-preservative sensitivity

Diagnosis

Superior epithelial arcuate lesion (SEAL)

Management

Contact lens wear was discontinued until the lesion healed. Unpreserved artificial tears were dispensed, to be used every hour. When the patient was reexamined in 3 days, the lesion was largely healed. After 6 days, the lesion was completely healed. The patient was then advised to return to daily disposable lens wear until a flatter base curve becomes available in the PureVision lens.

Discussion

The superior epithelial arcuate lesion, sometimes referred to as *epithelial splitting*, is a mechanical complication of soft lens wear, caused by extended wear of tight-fitting lenses.[1-4] It results from chronic indentation of the superior peripheral cornea by the peripheral curve junctions of a soft lens, which explains its parallel orientation to the limbus.[3] This is exacerbated by lenses with greater peripheral thickness and higher modulus. Tight upper eyelids contribute to the formation of this condition by pressing the lens periphery into the cornea. With long-term wear, the epithelium of the superior cornea undergoes mechanical irritation and begins to break down. The adjacent conjunctiva becomes injected, and in some cases, the patient notes mild to moderate pain. Although noninflammatory in nature, epithelial hypertrophy may result, giving the lesion a heaped-up appearance. Because of the epithelial defect, the lesion stains with fluorescein. In long-term cases, vascularization into the area may occur, leaving a pannus-like appearance on resolution.

Management of SEALs begins with discontinuation of lens wear. Topical antibiotics are usually unnecessary. Topical lubricants help reduce the patient's symptoms. The lesion usually resolves within 1–2 weeks. After resolution, the patient should be refitted to prevent recurrence. Changing lens design to one with a thinner periphery or changing the material to one with a lower modulus usually solves the problem. Flatter base curves help alleviate the peripheral compression. Finally, extended wear must be discontinued.

The patient was a questionable candidate for the PureVision lens due to his flat corneas and tight upper eyelids. It is not surprising that the lens periphery compressed the cornea and eventually resulted in this condition. In this case, despite a small amount of lens movement on blink, presumably allowed by the stiff lens material, the lens still proved to be too tight. In addition, this condition developed despite the high oxygen permeability of the lens, which indicates that hypoxia is not a major factor in its formation.[4]

The silicone hydrogel soft lens provides wearers with many advantages, but it must still be fitted and followed up carefully to detect potential complications.

Clinical Pearls

- SEALs are epithelial lesions that form parallel to the limbus.
- Tight-fitting relationships, thick lens periphery designs, and high lens modulus contribute to the formation of SEALs.
- Extended-wear patients with flat corneas and tight upper eyelids are more likely to develop SEALs.
- SEALs are noninflammatory and can be managed with lens discontinuation and artificial tears.

References

1. Davis LJ, Lebow KA. Non-infectious corneal staining. In: Silbert JA (ed). *Anterior Segment Complications of Contact Lens Wear*, 2nd ed. Boston: Butterworth–Heinemann, 2000:83.
2. Malinovsky V, Pole J, Pence NA, et al. Epithelial splits of the superior cornea in hydrogel contact lens patients. *Int Contact Lens Clin.* 1989;16(9):252–255.
3. Young G, Mirejovsky D. A hypothesis for the aetiology of soft contact lens-induced superior arcuate keratopathy. *Int Contact Lens Clin.* 1993;20(9):177–179.
4. Holden BA, Stephenson A, Stretton S, et al. Superior epithelial arcuate lesions with soft contact lens wear. *Optom Vis Sci.* 2001;78(1):9–12.

Soft Lens Discomfort

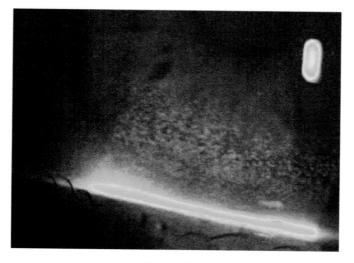

Figure 3-3

History

Patient AB is a 35-year-old Caucasian female who has been wearing ionic, high-water-content hydrogel disposable contact lenses (CL) on a daily-wear basis for the past 6 years. Her average wearing time is 14 hours per day, and she disposes of each pair of lenses on a monthly basis. Her current lenses are 3 weeks old. She uses a multipurpose solution to clean and disinfect her lenses daily, but she does not use an enzymatic cleaner. She also uses rewetting drops occasionally, when her eyes feel dry and irritated. Lately, her eyes have been feeling more irritated than usual when wearing her lenses. Her medical history is unremarkable. She takes oral contraceptives. She presently complains of mild dryness and irritation for the past few months, especially at work. She is an accountant and works on a computer most of the day.

Symptoms

- Mild dryness and irritation after 2–3 hours of wear for the past 2–3 months
- Mild conjunctival redness
- Decreased wear time

Clinical Data

- Entering visual acuity with CL:
  OD 20/20
  OS 20/20
- Contact lens specifications:
  OD Acuvue 8.8 / 14.0 / –1.75
  OS Acuvue 8.8 / 14.0 / –1.50
- Over-refraction: OU Plano sphere, 20/20
- Contact lens fit assessment: OU Slight superior-temporal position with full coverage, 0.25 mm movement on blink, mild protein film
- Keratometry:
  OD 43.75 / 44.00 @ 090
  OS 44.00 sphere
- Subjective refraction:
  OD –1.75 sphere, 20/20
  OS –1.50 sphere, 20/20
- Gross external exam: Interpalpebral injection OU: Grade 1 to 2
- Biomicroscopy: Grade 1 to 2 arcuate, inferior-central corneal epithelial punctate staining OU (see Figure 3-3)

Develop your list of differential diagnoses. Then, based on the clinical data, determine your final diagnosis. Based on your diagnosis, develop your treatment plan.

Differential Diagnoses

- Soft lens desiccation
- Giant papillary conjunctivitis
- Soft lens spoliation
- Preservative sensitivity
- Mechanical staining
- Viral conjunctivitis

Diagnosis

Soft lens desiccation

Management

The patient was refit to Proclear Compatibles soft lenses:

OD 8.6 / 14.2 / –1.75
OS 8.6 / 14.2 / –1.50

She was also instructed to use rewetting drops as needed when her eyes felt dry, especially at work. On follow-up visits, her symptoms were reduced markedly, although still present to a mild degree. Her corneal staining was reduced to trace amounts in each eye.

Discussion

Soft lens desiccation is a common finding among contact lens wearers. The diagnosis can usually be made from a thorough case history.[1] Although symptoms of irritation and dryness are often vague, careful probing can sometimes elicit complaints of a sandy or gritty sensation. Wearing time is also important to investigate. Patients usually start the day relatively comfortably, but as the day wears on, the lens dehydrates and progressively desiccates the eye. Older lenses usually have protein build-up, which causes them to dry out more quickly. Low-humidity climates and indoor environments also contribute to rapid lens drying.[2] Finally, people who do lots of near work, such as reading and computer work, tend to blink less frequently, which accelerates lens drying.

Ocular conditions such as the tear dysfunctions, blepharitis, and keratitis sicca also may cause dry eyes, which cause faster lens drying.[3] Certain systemic diseases, such as Sjögren's syndrome or rheumatoid arthritis, may contribute to dry eyes as well. Further, certain medications, such as antihistamines and oral contraceptives, may reduce tear production.

As a soft lens dehydrates, it draws water from the post-lens tear film, resulting in dryness of the cornea in these areas. Superficial punctate erosions then develop in the area of greatest dryness, which tends to be the interpalpebral inferior central zone of the cornea. This postlens dryness occurs more quickly and severely with thin, high-water-content designs.[4,5] Desiccation may be retarded by increasing lens thickness, using a low water content, or using materials that tend to dehydrate less.[6] Adjunct treatments include rewetting drops, although their benefit is usually short-lived.[7,8] Punctal occlusion has been found to be effective in certain patients with aqueous deficiencies.[9] In addition, any underlying lid disease, such as blepharitis or meibomitis, may cause a decrease in tear film quality and should be addressed prior to making any changes in contact lenses or adding any adjunct therapy.[3]

In this case, the patient's symptomatology points toward dry eye as the main problem. Her symptoms are bilateral and occur during working hours when she uses a computer for many hours. In addition, she takes a medication that tends to increase ocular dryness. Giant papillary conjunctivitis can be ruled out by performing lid eversion and inspecting the upper palpebral conjunctiva for papillae and inflammation. The contact lenses are slightly soiled, but her symptoms seem to be increasing despite a monthly replacement schedule, suggesting that soiled lenses are not the primary problem. Preservative sensitivity can occur after several months to years of successful solution use, but the symptoms would tend toward burning and stinging and occur soon after lens insertion, not late in the day. Viral conjunctivitis does not seem consistent with the patient's symptoms of increased discomfort at work and with the findings of interpalpebral (not diffuse) conjunctival injection.

Clinical Pearls

- Soft lenses that lower the rate of lens dehydration can significantly reduce symptoms of dryness.
- The underlying causes of tear film instability should be addressed prior to refitting.
- Adjunct therapies for dry eye include rewetting drops, frequent lens replacement, and punctal occlusion.

References

1. Orsborn G, Robboy M. Hydrogel lenses and dry-eye symptoms. *J Br Contact Lens Assoc.* 1989;11(6):37.
2. Andrasko G. Hydrogel dehydration in various environments. *Int Contact Lens Clin.* 1983;10(1):22.
3. Farris RL. Contact lenses and the dry eye. *Int Ophthalmol Clin.* 1994;34(1):129–136.
4. Orsborn GN, Zantos SG. Corneal desiccation staining with thin high water content contact lenses. *CLAO J.* 1988;14(2):81–85.
5. Little SA, Bruce AS. Role of the post-lens tear film in the mechanism of inferior arcuate staining with ultrathin hydrogel lenses. *CLAO J.* 1995;21(3):175–181.
6. Brennan NA, Efron N. Hydrogel lens dehydration: A material-dependent phenomenon? *Contact Lens Forum.* 1987;12(4):28.

7. Efron N, Golding TR, Brennan NA. The effect of soft lens lubricants on symptoms and lens dehydration. *CLAO J.* 1991;17(2):114–119.

8. Lowther GE. *Dryness, Tears and Contact Lens Wear.* Boston: Butterworth–Heinemann, 1997.

9. Slusser TG, Lowther GE. Effects of lacrimal drainage occlusion with nondissolvable intracanalicular plugs on hydrogel contact lens wear. *Optom Vis Sci.* 1998;75(5):330–338.

Redness with Rigid Gas-Permeable Lenses

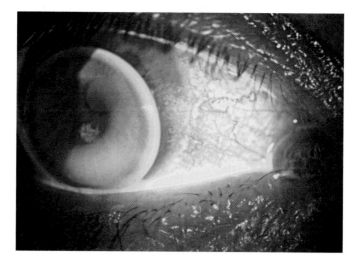

Figure 3-4

History

Patient BR, a 45-year-old Caucasian male, complains of redness and moderate irritation with his rigid gas-permeable (RGP) contact lenses (CL). He has keratoconus, for which he has worn RGP lenses for the past 20 years. His new symptoms began 2 weeks ago. They worsen as the day goes on but get better after he removes his lenses. The redness and irritation usually resolve by the next morning. However, it has gotten to the point that he is very concerned about the health of his eyes. Other than keratoconus, his ocular and medical histories are unremarkable. His current wearing time is 16 hours per day. He uses the Boston Original care system on a daily basis.

Symptoms

- Moderate bulbar injection in both eyes
- Moderate irritation in both eyes, worse as the day goes on

Clinical Data

- Entering visual acuity with CL:
  OD 20/20
  OS 20/15
- CL prescription:
  OD Polycon II / 7.40 / –3.25 / 9.5
  OS Boston RXD / 7.70 / –2.00 / 9.6
- CL evaluation:
  OD Inferior position, 1 mm movement, light three-point touch, surface clean with good wettability
  OS Central position, 2 mm movement, apical clearance with good peripheral clearance
- Gross external exam: Grade 3 interpalpebral injection OU, negative preauricular adenopathy
- Biomicroscopy: Moderate (grade 3) coalesced punctate staining interpalpebrally in the peripheral cornea OU, mild apical staining OD, faint striae centrally OD (see Figure 3-4)
- Keratometry (from topography):
  OD 46.10 @ 150 / 43.20 @ 070
  OS 45.48 @ 180 / 44.87 @ 090
- Subjective refraction:
  OD –1.25 –3.50 × 080, 20/30
  OS –3.00 –0.50 × 105, 20/20

Develop your list of differential diagnoses. Then, based on the clinical data, determine your final diagnosis. Based on your diagnosis, develop your treatment plan.

Differential Diagnoses

- Corneal abrasion
- Rigid lens desiccation
- Giant papillary conjunctivitis
- Discomfort from soiled lenses
- Preservative sensitivity
- Viral conjunctivitis
- Allergic conjunctivitis

Diagnosis

Rigid lens desiccation (3 and 9 o'clock staining)

Management

A solution preservative reaction was ruled out initially by changing the care system to one with a different preservative system. Because this did not reduce the signs and symptoms, corneal desiccation was diagnosed. The next treatment strategy was to redesign the RGP lenses with a smaller diameter. In addition, the material was changed to FluoroPerm 30 to increase wettability and Dk. Despite these lens changes and profuse rewetting, the staining persisted.

A piggyback system was then attempted with an Acuvue disposable lens and the same RGP lens. This reduced the patient's symptoms and the corneal staining significantly. However, the symptoms remained noticeable, so the piggyback system was discarded and punctal occlusion performed. The use of collagen diagnostic punctal plugs improved the symptoms, so silicone plugs were inserted. The patient was able to return to full-time rigid lens wear using extensive lubrication. Currently, the patient limits lens wear time when possible.

Discussion

Rigid lens desiccation is a common finding associated with RGP wear. In many cases, it is mild and needs only to be monitored.[1,2] However, in moderate to severe cases, it can create significant symptoms of redness and discomfort. This patient has moderate signs and symptoms associated with a dry eye. The contact lens in this case exacerbated the condition due to its fitting characteristics. A low-riding, immobile rigid contact lens tends to cause more extreme cases of peripheral desiccation by eliciting poor blinking habits and poor circulation of the tear film over the exposed areas.[3] The upper lid is averse to blinking over the superior edge of the lens, thereby creating incomplete and infrequent blinks. Even when the upper lid does blink, the edges of the lens hold the lid slightly away from the corneal surface adjacent to the lens edge, so the areas near 3 and 9 o'clock do not rewet properly. Therefore, the epithelial cells in this area dry out and subsequently stain positively with fluorescein. In addition, the adjacent interpalpebral conjunctiva becomes injected in response to dryness and the corneal response.[4]

Initially, this staining pattern may appear to be caused by a rigid lens abrasion. However, close examination reveals that the staining is outside the lens edge, which points to a different etiology.[5] If the staining were under the lens edge, a sharp edge or peripheral curve junction might be the causative factor. Of the other possible diagnoses, giant papillary conjunctivitis and discomfort from soiled lenses can be ruled out easily by everting the upper lids and ordering new lenses. A preservative sensitivity would cause a more diffuse injection and staining pattern. Although less common than before, due to formulations less irritating to the eye, this can still occur. Changing solution systems to those containing other preservatives rules this out. In this case, other solutions were tried with no improvement in symptoms.

The various forms of conjunctivitis must also be ruled out before settling on a diagnosis of peripheral desiccation. Since the condition is bilateral and mucous discharge is absent, bacterial conjunctivitis can be reasonably ruled out. Viral conjunctivitis is the most common variety and is often associated with an upper respiratory infection. Preauricular adenopathy, common to this condition, is absent in this case. Allergic conjunctivitis usually has itching as its primary symptom, and this is absent here. Removal of lenses alleviated all symptoms, which would not have occurred with an underlying conjunctivitis. Finally, conjunctivitis would more likely result in a diffuse conjunctival injection, not one that is limited to the interpalpebral space. Therefore, corneal desiccation is the most likely diagnosis.

This case is more challenging than most to manage because the patient has keratoconus. Keratoconus usually requires a rigid contact lens to provide clear vision. Therefore, a soft lens is usually not an option, even though it would alleviate the problems associated with peripheral desiccation. Other management options must be engaged. Changing care systems seems not to have helped. However, profuse lubrication throughout the day should be recommended. In mild cases, this is enough to alleviate symptoms. When symptomatology is greater, changes in lens material and design often help.[3,5] Changing to a mid-Dk fluorosilicone acrylate material enhances wettability. Changing the lens design to yield a more central or lid-attached position enhances lens movement and tear renewal over the epithelium. In this case, the lens material can be changed, but lens fit changes are limited by the keratoconus, which usually results in smaller designs that position inferiorly. Other contact lens options that can be utilized include hybrid (Soft-Perm) lenses and piggyback systems.

A final strategy is tear preservation via punctal occlusion. By maintaining a higher tear volume, the contact lens and ocular surface are less likely to dry out and cause symptoms. Punctal occlusion can be performed if lens design changes and rewetting drops alone do not alleviate the desiccation problem.

Clinical Pearl

- Rigid lens desiccation can be alleviated by lens design changes, extensive lubrication, and punctal occlusion.

References

1. Davis LJ, Lebow KA. Non-infectious corneal staining. In: Silbert JA (ed). *Anterior Segment Complications of Contact Lens Wear*, 2nd ed. Boston: Butterworth–Heinemann, 2000:73–77.
2. Jones DH, Bennett ES, Davis LJ. How to manage peripheral corneal desiccation. *Contact Lens Spectrum*. 1989;4(5):63.
3. Schnider CM, Terry RL, Holden BA. Effect of lens design on peripheral corneal desiccation. *J Am Optom Assoc*. 1997;68(3):163–170.
4. Schnider CM, Terry RL, Holden BA. Effect of patient and lens performance characteristics on peripheral corneal desiccation. *J Am Optom Assoc*. 1996;67(3):144–150.
5. Businger U, Treiber A, Flury C. The etiology and management of 3 and 9 o'clock staining. *Int Contact Lens Clin*. 1989;16(5):136.

More Redness with Rigid Gas-Permeable Lenses

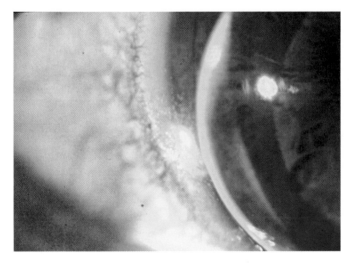

Figure 3-5

History

A 45-year-old Caucasian female complains of redness and irritation with her rigid gas-permeable (RGP) contact lenses (CL), OD more than OS. She has worn RGP contact lenses for the past 12 years. Her symptoms began several months ago and have steadily increased to where she is unable to wear her lenses for more than 2 hours. Her current pair of lenses is 2 years old. She normally wears them 14 hours per day and uses the Boston Advance Comfort Formula care system daily. Aside from these symptoms, her ocular history is unremarkable. Her medical history is significant for the use of Claritin D for seasonal allergies for the past year; otherwise, she is in good health.

Symptoms

Moderate redness and irritation, OD > OS with RGP lens wear

Clinical Findings

- Visual acuity with CL:
  OD 20/20
  OS 20/20
- CL prescription: Boston IV,
  OD 40.87 (8.26) / –2.50 / 9.4
  OS 41.00 (8.23) / –2.75 / 9.4
- CL evaluation: Inferior position, minimal movement, surface mildly protein-coated with poor wettability, apical alignment with mid-peripheral touch and minimal peripheral clearance OU
- Gross external exam: Interpalpebral injection OD grade 3, OS grade 2; negative preauricular adenopathy
- Biomicroscopy: White, elevated lesion with moderate (grade 3) coalesced punctate staining and neovascularization at 9 o'clock in the peripheral cornea OD (see Figure 3-5), mild (grade 2) 3 and 9 o'clock staining OU, no anterior chamber reaction
- Tear break-up time: 4 seconds OU
- Schirmer's test: 9 mm in 5 minutes OU

Develop your list of differential diagnoses. Then, based on the clinical data, determine your final diagnosis. Based on your diagnosis, develop your treatment plan.

Differential Diagnoses

- Corneal ulcer
- Inflamed pterygium
- Phlyctenulosis
- Rigid lens desiccation
- Viral conjunctivitis
- Allergic conjunctivitis

Diagnosis

Rigid lens desiccation (vascularized limbal keratitis, VLK)

Management

Lens wear was discontinued and the patient prescribed Polytrim drops q2h for the first day, then seen for a follow-up the next day. The dosage was then reduced to qid until the epithelial defect healed completely. At that point, the Polytrim was discontinued. Because the infiltrate was mild and neovascularization minimal, a steroid was not determined to be necessary. Instead, the patient was given artificial tears. After resolution of the infiltrate, the patient was refitted with the following RGP lenses:

OD FluoroPerm 30 / 8.05 / –2.50 / 8.7
OS FluoroPerm 30 / 8.05 / –2.50 / 8.7

These lenses showed a more central lens position with moderate peripheral clearance. On follow-up, the 3 and 9 o'clock staining returned to a mild degree. The patient was closely monitored for recurrence of the VLK. She continues to use the rewetting drops regularly.

Discussion

This case illustrates a severe manifestation of peripheral corneal desiccation from RGP wear. Vascularized limbal keratitis is caused by severe, chronic desiccation of the peripheral corneal epithelium that eventually stimulates epithelial hypertrophy, erosion, and neovascular vessel growth into the affected area.[1-3] In early stages, symptomatology is mild, similar to mild dry eye. In later stages, symptoms may suggest a sterile corneal ulcer. In fact, if an epithelial defect is present over the affected area, an ulcer should be suspected until proven otherwise.

Several factors of this case lead to the diagnosis of VLK. First, the interpalpebral injection and 3 and 9 o'clock staining in both eyes suggests an underlying, chronic dryness condition. Second, signs of frank corneal ulcer, such as localized injection, mucous discharge, and anterior chamber reaction, are absent. Third, the lesion does not have the appearance of a pterygium, which is a fibrovascular growth moving onto the cornea from the conjunctiva; instead, there is a clear zone between the lesion and the limbus. Phlyctenule is a possible diagnosis but, given the overall scenario, not as likely. Viral and allergic conjunctivitis are also less likely because of the lack of associated factors.

VLK should be treated as a potential precursor to a corneal ulcer. Since an epithelial defect is present, it must be covered with a broad spectrum antibiotic effective against gram-negative bacteria, such as *Pseudomonas*, as well as common gram-positives, such as *Staphylococcus*. Polytrim or Tobramycin drops are acceptable options. Additionally, the cloudy lesion can be treated with a steroid to accelerate resolution. A mild steroid, such as Vexol or Lotemax, or a combination drug, such as Tobradex, can be used. Once the lesion is resolved, the contact lens must be refit to prevent recurrence.[1-3] A central or lid-attached lens is less likely to cause desiccation. If a soft lens can provide acceptable visual acuity, one can be fitted. In extreme cases, options such as hybrid (Soft-Perm) lenses or piggyback systems can be used. In addition, dry eye therapy, such as extensive lubrication and punctal occlusion can be useful. Finally, the patient's medications should be investigated. If it is possible to eliminate the oral antihistamine, the patient's eyes would not be as dry. A delicate discussion of the decrease in tear production with age may also be warranted to assure the patient that her condition is normal.

Clinical Pearls

- Severe rigid lens desiccation can cause corneal lesions that resemble ulcers and other inflammatory conditions.
- Lesions with overlying epithelial defects must be treated prophylactically with antibiotics.
- Inflammatory lesions can be treated with topical steroids along with antibacterial coverage.
- Vascularized limbal keratitis has a dry eye etiology and requires long-term management.

References

1. Grohe RM, Lebow KA. Vascularized limbal keratitis. *Int Contact Lens Clin.* 1989;16(7):197.
2. Davis LJ, Lebow KA. Non-infectious corneal staining. In: Silbert JA (ed). *Anterior Segment Complications of Contact Lens Wear*, 2nd ed. Boston: Butterworth–Heinemann, 2000:77–81.
3. Edwards K, Hough T. Contact lens–related case studies: Vascularised limbal keratitis. *Optician.* 1998;216(5680):36–37.

Itchy Soft Lens

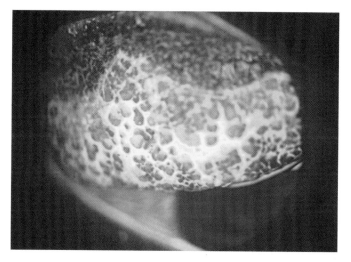

Figure 3-6

History

A 32-year-old Caucasian male complains of discomfort, itchiness, and mucous discharge with his current soft contact lenses (CL), OD more than OS. These symptoms began about 2 weeks ago and have worsened each day. He has worn conventional soft lenses for 15 years. His current pair is 2 years old. He uses AOSept with Ultrazyme to clean and disinfect his lenses. His current wearing time is 14 hours per day. His ocular and medical histories are unremarkable.

Symptoms

- Lens discomfort
- Itchiness
- Mucous discharge

Clinical Data

- Visual acuity with CL:
  OD 20/30
  OS 20/20
- CL prescription: B&L Soflens U4, OD –9.00, OS –8.50
- Over-refraction:
  OD Plano –0.25 × 180, 20/30
  OS Plano sphere, 20/20
- Lens fit assessment: Centered OU, movement on blink 2 mm OD and 0.5 mm OS, surface protein deposition grade 3 OD and grade 1 OS
- External examination: No preauricular adenopathy noted
- Biomicroscopy: Bulbar injection grade 1 OU; diffuse corneal staining grade 2 OD and grade 1 OS; neovascularization grade 2 OU; tarsal papillae and hyperemia grade 3 OD and grade 1 OS (see Figure 3-6); white, ropy mucous discharge OD > OS
- Keratometry:
  OD 44.50 / 44.75 @ 80, grade 1 distortion
  OS 43.75 / 44.25 @ 90, no distortion
- Subjective refraction:
  OD –10.25 –0.25 × 175, 20/40
  OS –9.50 sphere, 20/25

Develop your list of differential diagnoses. Then, based on the clinical data, determine your final diagnosis. Based on your diagnosis, develop your treatment plan.

Differential Diagnoses

- Giant papillary conjunctivitis
- Vernal conjunctivitis
- Viral conjunctivitis
- Atopic keratoconjunctivitis
- Adult inclusion conjunctivitis

Diagnosis

Giant papillary conjunctivitis (GPC)

Management

Because this patient was a high myope and had no glasses, it was not possible to immediately discontinue lens wear. He was refit temporarily with disposable soft lenses and given a spectacle prescription to fill immediately. He was to discontinue lens wear and return in 1 week. He was given artificial tears to use every 2–3 hours. A topical therapeutic agent was deemed unnecessary because his symptoms were much reduced after lens removal. After approximately 3 weeks of no lens wear, the patient was refitted to 1-week disposable lenses. He was educated on the causes of his GPC as well as proper lens care and replacement schedules to prevent future episodes.

Discussion

Although this clinical picture can be due to many different clinical entities, several factors point to soft lens–induced GPC. First, there is no history of systemic allergies or other atopic conditions, and the patient is not in the age range typical for vernal conjunctivitis. Next, the lack of preauricular adenopathy and the presence of a white, ropy mucous discharge suggest something other than a viral etiology. Although chlamydia is a possibility, it is much less likely to be the cause, considering the presence of soiled lenses, which is the most common cause of GPC.

GPC is a combined mechanical and immune response to denatured surface proteins.[1-3] The proteins create a roughened surface that mechanically irritates the superior palpebral conjunctiva. In addition, there is a delayed hypersensitivity response to the proteins, which become foreign to the immune system after they become denatured. The condition begins with mild discomfort and tarsal hyperemia. As it progresses, large papillae form on the upper tarsus, and increased mucous discharge, itchiness, and irritation develop. In severe stages, lens wear becomes intolerable. Excessive lens movement is also common as friction between the roughened palpebral conjunctiva and the roughened lens surface increases.

This condition should not be confused with tarsal papillary hypertrophy, which can occur for other reasons and is usually asymptomatic. With papillary hypertrophy, large papillae are present on the upper tarsus, but they usually occur near the tarsal fold without hyperemia.[1,3] In addition, patients have no symptoms as described here. Large papillae may not be present in the early stages of GPC, but symptoms always exist to some degree.

Treatment begins with discontinuation of lens wear, if possible.[1-6] In mild to moderate cases, immediate refitting is a viable option if the patient has good comfort with new lenses.[4] This patient had high myopia and no spectacles. This is a common problem, but the patient must be informed of the reasons for having a pair of glasses to wear when he is unable to wear contact lenses. Temporarily, disposable trial lenses can be dispensed so that he can get home safely. The ultimate goal is to allow the patient to continue healthy lens wear. Disposable lenses are a good option because of frequent lens replacement and expanded parameters for high myopia, hyperopia, astigmatism, and presbyopia.[5] Protein-resistant materials should be utilized, if possible.[2-4,6] In addition, an unpreserved care system with separate daily cleaner is recommended. In extreme cases, enzymatic cleaning of the disposable lenses can be added. If soft lenses fail, even with these strategies, RGP lenses may be required.

Medical therapy is dictated by signs and symptoms. In mild to moderate cases, artificial tears or mild topical medications, such as antihistamines or nonsteroidal anti-inflammatory drugs, can be used on a qid basis. In severe cases, topical steroids may be required to alleviate symptoms. Because this is an ocular surface condition, steroids with good ocular penetration are not necessary. "Soft steroids," such as loteprednol and rimexolone, are good options for GPC and have fewer unwanted side effects.[2-4,6]

Clinical Pearls

- GPC does not always have large papillae on the upper tarsus.
- Large papillae on the upper tarsus are not always caused by GPC.
- Immediate refitting into new lenses can be a viable treatment for mild to moderate GPC.
- Disposable lenses are good first options for previous soft lens wearers.
- RGP lenses may be necessary in recalcitrant cases.
- Medical management may be necessary in severe cases.

References

1. Allansmith MR, Korb DR, Greiner JV. Giant papillary conjunctivitis in contact lens wearers. *Am J Ophthalmol.* 1977; 83(5):697–708.
2. Katelaris CH. Giant papillary conjunctivitis—A review. *Acta Ophthalmol Scand.* 1999; 77(228):17–20.

3. Jurkus JM. Contact lens–induced giant papillary conjunctivitis. In: Silbert JA (ed). *Anterior Segment Complications of Contact Lens Wear*, 2nd ed. Boston: Butterworth–Heinemann, 2000:133–148.
4. Schultz JE. Treating giant papillary conjunctivitis while wearing contact lenses. *Int Contact Lens Clin.* 1990;17(5):139–143.
5. Porazinski AD, Donshik PC. Giant papillary conjunctivitis in frequent replacement contact lens wearers: A retrospective study. *CLAO J.* 1999;25(3):142–147.
6. Lazarou ZK. Contact lens–associated giant papillary conjunctivitis. *Clin Eye Vis Care.* 1999;11(1):33–35.

Itchy Rigid Gas-Permeable Lens

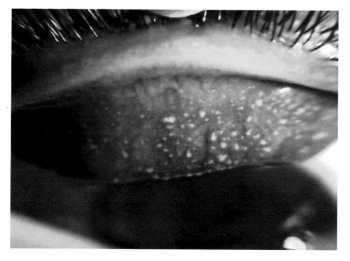

Figure 3-7

History

Patient EO, an 18-year-old Hispanic male, presents with symptoms of discomfort, itchiness, and stringy mucous discharge OD more than OS, for the past month. He reports that he has had to decrease his wearing time from 14 to 6 hours per day. He is a 4-year rigid gas-permeable (RGP) contact lenses (CL) wearer. His current lenses are 3 years old. He uses the Boston Original care system daily. He has a history of mild tarsal papillae and blepharitis, for which he occasionally does warm compresses and lid scrubs. Otherwise, his ocular and medical histories are unremarkable.

Symptoms

- Lens discomfort
- Itchiness
- Stringy mucous discharge

Clinical Data

- Visual acuity with CL:
  OD 20/20 (slow)
  OS 20/15
- CL prescription: Boston ES,
  OD 8.10 / –1.75 / 9.6
  OS 8.10 / –2.00 / 9.6
- Over-refraction:
  OD Plano sphere, 20/20
  OS Plano sphere, 20/15
- Lens fit assessment: Superior-central with lid attachment, 2 mm movement on blink OU; apical and mid-peripheral alignment, moderate peripheral clearance OU; grade 1 protein and moderate scratches on lens surface OU
- Keratometry:
  OD 42.00 / 42.50 @ 090
  OS 41.75 / 42.50 @ 090
- Subjective refraction:
  OD –2.00 sphere, 20/15
  OS –2.50 sphere, 20/15
- Biomicroscopy: Upper tarsus, grade 3 large papillae with scarring OD (see Figure 3-7), grade 1 to 2 papillae OS; mild crusting of eyelashes OU; all other structures clear and healthy OU

Develop your list of differential diagnoses. Then, based on the clinical data, determine your final diagnosis. Based on your diagnosis, develop your treatment plan.

Differential Diagnoses

- Giant papillary conjunctivitis
- Vernal conjunctivitis
- Viral conjunctivitis
- Adult inclusion conjunctivitis

Diagnosis

RGP contact lens–induced giant papillary conjunctivitis (GPC)

Management

Contact lens wear was discontinued and Patanol ophthalmic solution prescribed bid for the right eye for 4 weeks. The patient returned 2 months later for a contact lens refitting. He reported complete resolution of symptoms. Biomicroscopy revealed grade 1–2 tarsal papillae with scarring OD and grade 1 tarsal papillae OS. The patient was then refitted with Focus Dailies soft disposable lenses to eliminate all lens care and the potential for developing deposits that would reactivate the GPC. The patient returned 5 months later for a complete eye exam and wanted to return to RGP lenses due to the high cost of daily disposable lenses. New RGP lenses were ordered and dispensed. The patient was reeducated on proper lens care with the Boston Original care system and Boston Liquid Enzyme. He was advised to return in 6 months for a progress evaluation.

Discussion

Although GPC is typically associated with soft lens wear, it can also be caused by RGP lenses.[1] RGP lenses can become coated with denatured proteins just as soft lenses can, especially with poorly wetting lenses and improper lens care.[2–5] In addition, because GPC is caused by mechanical as well as immunological stimuli, any edge or surface irregularity that causes excessive mechanical trauma to the upper tarsus can induce GPC.[2] This is evidenced by cases of GPC caused by suture barbs and ocular prostheses.

The clinical picture of RGP-induced GPC is often different from that of soft lens–induced GPC. The papillary response is usually localized to a smaller area, closer to the lid margin (zone 3).[2,6] This is the area of the tarsus that comes into contact with the lens most frequently. This pattern of papillary hypertrophy is not found with soft lens–induced GPC or vernal conjunctivitis.

However, symptoms can be quite similar between RGP- and soft lens–induced GPC.[1–6] Itchiness, lens discomfort, and ropy mucous discharge all are hallmarks. Because the ocular response is the same regardless of the etiological agent, the treatment is similar.

Lens discontinuation is usually required to give the patient's eyelid time to heal. Artificial tears, antihistamines, mast cell stabilizers, nonsteroidal anti-inflammatory drugs, or steroids can be used, based on the severity of symptoms and signs.[2] On resolution of symptoms, a new lens with an optimal edge design should be ordered.[7] Daily disposable soft lenses are another good option, especially for noncompliant patients. However, patients accustomed to the sharp visual acuity and durability of RGP lenses may not be as satisfied with soft lenses.

To optimize the edge design of an RGP lens, edge thickness and shape must be specified. Edge thickness should be 0.10–0.12 mm prior to finishing. High minus powers and lid-attachment designs use greater edge thicknesses, which lead to greater interaction with the upper lid. Edge shape should be slightly rounded, with the apex at or slightly behind the geometric center of the edge. An apex too far forward may irritate the upper lid. Finally, edge lift should be specified for the best balance between comfort and lid interaction. A lower edge lift is more comfortable, but a higher edge lift enhances lid attachment. An edge lift of 0.10–0.16 mm provides most patients with good comfort and sufficient lid attachment.

Lens care is of great importance, too. A daily cleaner that is also abrasive, such as Boston Cleaner or Alcon OptiSoak Cleaner, helps remove hard protein films. Regular use of an enzymatic cleaner, such as Boston Liquid Enzyme or Alcon Supraclens, also helps keep the lens surface clean.[8] Finally, patient education on proper lens care and the importance of routine follow-up visits go a long way in preventing recurrence of this patient's contact lens problem.

Clinical Pearls

- GPC can be caused by RGP lenses.
- RGP-induced GPC can be deposit related or mechanical in nature.
- Medical management of RGP-induced GPC is similar to that of soft lens–induced GPC.
- Edge integrity and design are important in preventing GPC.
- Proper lens care is important in preventing protein surface deposits and GPC.

References

1. Korb DR, Allansmith MR, Greiner JV, et al. Prevalence of conjunctival changes in wearers of hard contact lenses. *Am J Ophthalmol.* 1980;90(3):336–341.

2. Jurkus JM. Contact lens–induced giant papillary conjunctivitis. In: Silbert JA (ed). *Anterior Segment Complications of Contact Lens Wear*, 2nd ed. Boston: Butterworth–Heinemann, 2000:133–148.

3. Allansmith MR, Korb DR, Greiner JV, et al. Giant papillary conjunctivitis in contact lens wearers. *Am J Ophthalmol.* 1977;83:697.

4. Schnider CM. Rigid gas-permeable extended-wear lenses. In: Silbert JA (ed). *Anterior Segment Complications of Contact Lens Wear*, 2nd ed. Boston: Butterworth–Heinemann, 2000:315–316.

5. Fowler SA, Korb DR, Finnemore VM, et al. Surface deposits on worn hard contact lenses. *Arch Ophthalmol.* 1984; 102(5):757–759.

6. Korb DR, Allansmith MR, Greiner JV, et al. Biomicroscopy of papillae associated with hard contact lens wearing. *Ophthalmol.* 1981;88(11):1132–1136.

7. Roy A. Management of contact lens–associated papillary conjunctivitis using gas-permeable contact lenses. *J Brit Contact Lens Assoc.* 1994;17(1):7–10.

8. Korb DR, Greiner JV, Finnemore VM, et al. Treatment of contact lenses with papain. Increase in wearing time in keratoconic patients with papillary conjunctivitis. *Arch Ophthalmol.* 1983;101(1):48–50.

Soft Lens Discomfort

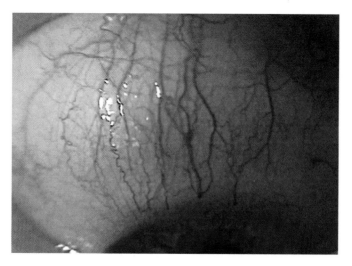

Figure 3-8

History

A 29-year-old Caucasian female complains of redness and irritation in her right eye for the past month. Her eyes also feel dry, and she uses rewetting drops, which provide some relief. Discontinuing lens wear reduces her symptoms, but resumption of lens wear causes the symptoms to return. She wears conventional soft lenses and wears them 12 hours each day. She has worn soft lenses for 10 years, and her current lenses are almost 2 years old. She uses "store brand" solutions to clean and disinfect her lenses. Further questioning reveals that she switches from brand to brand depending on store sales. Her ocular and medical histories are otherwise unremarkable. She reports taking oral contraceptives but has no known allergies. She presents today wearing her glasses.

Symptoms

- Unilateral redness and irritation with soft lens wear
- Symptoms are reduced, but not eliminated, with discontinuation of lens wear

Clinical Data

- VA with spectacles:
  OD 20/25^{-2}
  OS 20/20
- Keratometry:
  OD 45.50 / 46.00 @ 083, clear mires
  OS 46.50 / 46.00 @ 083, clear mires
- Subjective refraction
  OD −5.50 −0.50 × 010, 20/20
  OS −4.25 −0.50 × 030, 20/20
- Biomicroscopy:
  OD: Grade 3 superior bulbar injection (see Figure 3-8); grade 2 tarsal papillary hypertrophy; grade 2 superior corneal staining; grade 1 neovascularization superiorly; anterior chamber quiet
  OS: Grade 2 tarsal papillary hypertrophy, grade 1 neovascularization superiorly; anterior chamber quiet
- CL prescription: Cibasoft,
  OD 8.6 / 13.8 / −5.25
  OS 8.6 / 13.8 / −4.25
- Lens inspection: Grade 2 protein film OU

Develop your list of differential diagnoses. Then, based on the clinical data, determine your final diagnosis. Based on your diagnosis, develop your treatment plan.

Differential Diagnoses

- Giant papillary conjunctivitis
- Solution preservative sensitivity
- Superior limbic keratoconjunctivitis
- Simple episcleritis

Diagnosis

Contact lens–induced superior limbic keratoconjunctivitis (CL-SLK)

Management

Lens wear was discontinued until the redness and irritation resolved. Artificial tears were prescribed for use every 2 hours in the affected eye. The patient returned 1 week later with resolution of signs and symptoms. At this visit, a disposable soft lens was refitted:

Proclear Compatibles / 8.6 / 14.2 / –5.25 and –4.25
Visual acuity with CL: OD 20/20, OS 20/20
Fit assessment: Centered, 1 mm movement on blink, good lag

The patient appreciated clear vision and good comfort. Her wear time was gradually increased to 14 hours per day. She was given QuickCare to clean and disinfect her lenses and instructed to replace her lens every month. She noted no problems at her 1-month follow-up visit.

Discussion

The localization of the bulbar injection and corneal staining to the superior quadrant are the biggest clues to making this diagnosis. Other factors leading to this diagnosis include the soiled contact lenses and tarsal papillary response. The contact lens–induced version of SLK, in most cases, is an immunological response to a contact lens with significant protein coating or a preservative like thimerosal.[1-3] A tarsal response often is associated with this form of SLK, although often less intense than in Theodore's SLK.[1,2]

A solution preservative allergy alone would manifest as bilateral, diffuse redness and itchiness, which is not the pattern in this case. Episcleritis is a possibility, but because symptoms are reduced when the lenses are removed, a contact lens etiology is suggested.

CL-SLK should be differentiated from the Theodore's form of SLK. Theodore's SLK is not contact lens related but can be associated with hyperthyroidism. It also tends to occur in 20–50 year olds, is more prevalent in women, and is usually bilateral. Finally, it tends to come and go over a 5- to 10-year period.[1-4]

Treatment of CL-SLK begins with discontinuation of lens wear. Topical therapies, such as vasoconstrictors, nonsteroidal anti-inflammatory drugs, and steroids, can be helpful in severe cases, but preservative-free artificial tears usually suffice.[1,2] Once the condition resolves, refitting with disposable lenses with low water content and nonionic surfaces is recommended. A change to a nonpreserved care system is also recommended.[1,2] Although not common today, thimerosal is still found in inexpensive saline solutions. The patient's history of using various generic brands may include using a thimerosal-preserved solution. With old, protein-coated lenses, these irritating preservatives may adhere to the lens surface, which would increase the contact time of the preservative with the ocular surface, inducing this response. Clean lenses that are disinfected with unpreserved solutions are less likely to cause a recurrence.

Clinical Pearls

- CL-SLK should be differentiated from Theodore's SLK.
- CL-SLK can be caused by solution preservatives or soiled lenses.
- Thimerosal is a common cause of CL-SLK and can still be found in certain solutions.

References

1. Abel R, Shovlin JP, DePaolis MD. A treatise on hydrophilic lens induced superior limbic keratoconjunctivitis. *Int Contact Lens Clin.* 1985;12(2):116–123.
2. Silbert JA. Diagnostic dilemmas: Contact lens–induced SLK vs. Theodore's SLK. *Rev Optom.* 1996;133(4):95–96.
3. Sendele DD, Kenyon KR, Mobilia EF, et al. Superior limbic keratoconjunctivitis in contact lens wearers. *Opthalmol.* 1983; 90(6):616–622.
4. Fuerst DJ, Sugar J, Worobec S. Superior limbic keratoconjunctivitis associated with cosmetic soft contact lens wear. *Arch Ophthalmol.* 1983;101(8):1214–1216.

CASE 3-9

Routine Soft Lens Wearer

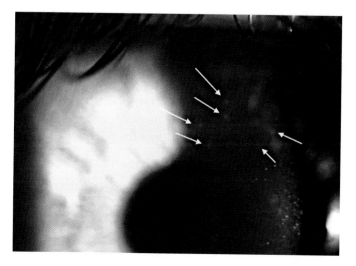

Figure 3-9

History

A 23-year-old Caucasian female presents for a routine eye examination. She reports good vision and has no ocular complaints. She has been a disposable soft lens wearer for the past 4 years and wears her lenses 15 hours a day. She uses Complete multipurpose solution to clean and disinfect her lenses. Her ocular and medical histories are unremarkable. She takes no medications but has an allergy to amoxicillin.

Symptoms

No symptoms were reported

Clinical Data

- Entering visual acuity with CL:
  OD 20/20
  OS 20/20–
- CL prescription: Soflens 66, unknown parameters
- Contact lens fit: OU centered, 1 mm movement on blink, clean lens surfaces
- External exam: Unremarkable OU
- Keratometry:
  OD 43.50 sphere
  OS 43.25 / 43.75 @ 090
- Subjective refraction:
  OD –4.00 sphere, 20/20
  OS –3.75 sphere, 20/20–
- Biomicroscopy: Grade 1 conjunctival injection OU; several pinpoint subepithelial infiltrates scattered diffusely OU (see Figure 3-9); grade 1 diffuse positive and negative corneal staining OU; all other structures appear clear and healthy OU

Develop your list of differential diagnoses. Then, based on the clinical data, determine your final diagnosis. Based on your diagnosis, develop your treatment plan.

Differential Diagnoses

- Infiltrative keratitis
- Corneal ulcer
- Solution preservation sensitivity
- Viral conjunctivitis
- Allergic conjunctivitis

Diagnosis

Infiltrates due to solution preservative sensitivity

Management

Lens wear was discontinued. The patient was prescribed Refresh Plus unpreserved tears every 2 hours. She was reexamined 3 weeks later. The infiltrates had resolved in her right eye but were still present in her left eye. Mild corneal staining was still present inferiorly. She continued the Refresh Plus and was instructed to return in 2 weeks. At this visit, the infiltrates were still present in her left eye, and trace corneal staining remained present inferiorly. Two weeks later, the infiltrates still remained in her left eye. She was started on Lotemax 0.5% drops qid OS only and instructed to return in 1 week. A week later, her infiltrates were gone and her staining had resolved. She was then fit with Pure Vision soft lenses, dispensed QuickCare for cleaning and disinfection, and told to return for a follow-up 2 weeks later. Her corneas were clear at the 2-week follow-up visit and remained clear 9 months later.

Discussion

Contact lens–induced infiltrates can result from soiled lenses, overwear, or reactions to solution preservatives.[1–5] In this case, the patient had persistent infiltrates associated with soft lens wear. She did not overwear her lenses and did not have dirty, soiled lenses. However, she used a multipurpose solution to clean and disinfect her lenses, so this was the most likely etiology of her infiltrates.[1,2] Early on, small corneal infiltrates may not produce appreciable symptoms.[1–7] A mild conjunctival injection was noted on biomicroscopy. Because of the relatively mild presentation of the infiltrates, it was not deemed necessary to treat aggressively with therapeutic agents. However, it is important to differentiate infectious versus noninfectious infiltrates.[6,7] Solution-related infiltrates usually resolve on their own once lens wear is ceased.[1,2] In this case, the right eye healed very quickly, but the left eye had persistent infiltrates. After several weeks of palliative treatment with unpreserved artificial tears and little resolution, a topical steroid was added to accelerate healing. Within a week of initiating steroid treatment, the infiltrates resolved. This indicates that immediate treatment of contact lens–related infiltrates with topical steroids would allow more rapid resolution. However, because other etiologies, such as an adenoviral or herpetic infection, must be ruled out prior to steroid treatment, it often is best to wait a few weeks to see how the cornea responds to discontinuation of lens wear alone. After several weeks and with an otherwise white and quiet eye, topical steroids can be confidently prescribed for persistent infiltrates. Once the infiltrates have resolved and the patient is ready to resume lens wear, an unpreserved care system should be prescribed.

Other potential causative factors in the development of corneal infiltrates are hypoxia and lens surface deposits. By increasing the Dk/L and deposit resistance of the contact lens, these two factors can be minimized. The PureVision is a silicone hydrogel lens with a Dk/L of

100. In addition, its surface is treated to resist surface deposits and bacteria adhesion. Although the treatment tends to degrade over the course of 2 or 3 months, for the recommended 1-month wearing cycle, it is very good at repelling deposits. In addition, by changing the care system to one with a separate daily cleaner, the patient has cleaner lens surfaces.

Clinical Pearls

- Corneal infiltrates can be induced by contact lens overwear, soiled lenses, or solution preservatives.
- Persistent infiltrates can be treated with a topical steroid.
- Viral and other infectious etiologies should be ruled out prior to initiation of topical steroid treatment.

References

1. Snyder C. Infiltrative keratitis with contact lens wear—A review. *J Am Optom Assoc.* 1995;66(3):160–177.
2. Yeung KK, Weissman BA. Presumed sterile corneal infiltrates and hydrogel lens wear: A case series. *Int Contact Lens Clin.* 1997;24(6):213–216.
3. Suchecki JK, Ehlers WH, Donshik PC. Peripheral corneal infiltrates associated with contact lens wear. *CLAO J.* 1996; 22(1):41–46.
4. Smay JC. Sterile corneal infiltrates: Differential diagnosis and clinical management. *Optom Today.* 1998;6(2):54–62.
5. Cutter GR, Chalmers RL, Roseman M. The clinical presentation, prevalence, and risk factors of focal corneal infiltrates in soft contact lens wearers. *CLAO J.* 1996;22(1):30–37.
6. Stein RM, Clinch TE, Cohen EJ, et al. Infected vs. sterile corneal infiltrates in contact lens wearers. *Am J Ophthalmol.* 1988; 105(6):632–636.
7. Cohen EJ. Management of small corneal infiltrates in contact lens wearers. *Arch Ophthalmol.* 2000;118(2):276–277.

"There's a White Spot on My Eye"

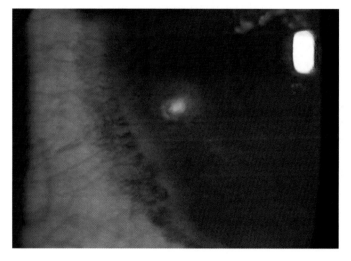

Figure 3-10

History

A 22-year-old Asian male complains of mild redness and irritation in his right eye for the past 3 days. He also notes a small white spot on his cornea. He does not report photophobia, discharge, or blurry vision. He currently wears soft contact lenses on a daily-wear basis with an average wearing time of 12 hours per day. He denies sleeping in his lenses. He uses Opti-Free for overnight soaking and Opti-Free Daily Cleaner to clean the lenses every 2–3 days. He replaces his lenses every 3 months. His current pair is 2 months old. He denies previous problems with contact lens wear. His ocular and medical histories are otherwise unremarkable. He takes no medications and has no allergies.

Symptoms

- Mild redness and irritation
- Small white spot on the cornea

Clinical Data

- Visual acuity with spectacles:
  OD 20/20–
  OS 20/20–
- CL prescription: Ciba Focus,
  OD 8.6 / 14.0 / –1.50
  OS 8.6 / 14.0 / –1.50
- Lens fit assessment: Centered, 0.5 mm movement OU; grade 1 protein film OU
- Keratometry:
  OD 42.00 sphere
  OS 42.00 sphere
- Subjective refraction:
  OD –1.50 sphere, 20/20
  OS –1.50 sphere, 20/20
- Pupils: PERRL-APD
- Biomicroscopy: Sectoral bulbar injection at 8 o'clock OD; positively staining white, cloudy lesion 1 mm in diameter at 8 o'clock in the corneal periphery, epithelial and anterior stromal, with surrounding haze OD (see Figure 3-10); grade 2 neovascularization superiorly OU; grade 1 diffuse punctate staining OU; grade 2 microcysts OU; anterior chamber quiet OU; lids clear OU

Develop your list of differential diagnoses. Then, based on the clinical data, determine your final diagnosis. Based on your diagnosis, develop your treatment plan.

Differential Diagnoses

- Microbial corneal ulcer
- Sterile corneal ulcer
- Pterygium
- Phlyctenule
- Vascularized limbal keratitis

Diagnosis

Sterile corneal ulcer

Management

Lens wear was discontinued. The patient was started on Ciloxan every hour in his right eye. He was reexamined 24 hours later, and the ulcer was unchanged. The antibiotic therapy was maintained for another day. The next day, the ulcer appeared to be resolving slightly, so the Ciloxan dosage was reduced to every 2 hours. The following day, the ulcer was reduced, although the epithelial defect and infiltrate were still present. The dosage was reduced to qid. One week later, the epithelial defect was almost gone, so the dosage was reduced to bid. The patient was instructed to return in 1 week, but did not return for 6 weeks. At that visit, the ulcer was healed, and a scar remained. It was recommended that he be refitted with rigid gas-permeable (RGP) contact lenses.

Discussion

This case illustrates a classic contact lens–induced peripheral corneal ulcer. The loss of epithelial and anterior stromal tissue constitutes an ulcer; however, the etiology of this ulcer is not microbial but immune. Most contact lens–induced corneal ulcers are culture negative, suggesting either that they are noninfectious or that current culturing procedures are inadequate to detect the microbes responsible.[1-6] Either way, most contact lens–induced ulcers begin as infiltrates, which erode the overlying epithelium. The immune response also manifests as bulbar injection and diffuse corneal haze consisting of white blood cells and stromal edema surrounding the primary lesion.[1-7] If left untreated, these "sterile" ulcers can become infected.

The differentiation of "sterile" and infectious ulcers can be difficult.[1,2,4-8] "Sterile" ulcers tend to be mildly irritating peripheral lesions less than 1 mm in diameter. Local injection is present, but there is a lack of mucous discharge, anterior chamber reaction, and lid involvement. Infectious ulcers tend to be painful, more centrally located, and greater than 1 mm in diameter. Patients usually have copious mucous discharge, diffuse injection, positive anterior chamber reaction, and lid edema.

Although most contact lens–induced ulcers are noninfectious, they should be treated as infectious unless found to be culture negative.[2,4,7] Current treatment includes fluoroquinolones q30min to qh for the first 24 hours, with follow-up the next day. Dosage is then adjusted according to the healing response. Once the epithelium has healed, a topical steroid can be added to aid resolution of the infiltrate. However, in almost all cases, a scar will remain.

After resolution, contact lens wear should be resumed with caution. The best option would be a high Dk, frequently replaced soft lens or an RGP. Currently, the silicone hydrogel contact lens has the highest available Dk. Worn on a daily wear basis, the lens provides more than enough oxygen to prevent compromise of corneal function. An RGP also provides adequate oxygen and has the advantage of better tear exchange and fewer surface deposits, both factors in the development of infiltrates. Nonpreserved hydrogen peroxide care systems are recommended for maximum disinfection of soft lenses while minimizing potential adverse effects from solution preservatives.[7]

Thorough patient education is crucial to prevent a second episode. Wearing time should be limited to daily wear, lenses must be cleaned properly on a daily basis, lenses should be replaced regularly, and the patient must return for routine examinations every 6–12 months.

Clinical Pearls

- It is important to differentiate noninfectious from infectious ulcers.
- The majority of contact lens–induced ulcers are noninfectious.
- Initial treatment of presumed noninfectious ulcers must assume infection is present.
- Current standard initial treatment of corneal ulcers is a topical fluoroquinolone.

References

1. Suchecki JK, Ehlers WH, Donshik PC. Peripheral corneal infiltrates associated with contact lens wear. *CLAO J.* 1996; 22(1):41–46.
2. Smay JC. Sterile corneal infiltrates: Differential diagnosis and clinical management. *Optom Today.* 1998;6(2):54–62.

3. Cutter GR, Chalmers RL, Roseman M. The clinical presentation, prevalence, and risk factors of focal corneal infiltrates in soft contact lens wearers. *CLAO J.* 1996;22(1):30–37.
4. Cohen EJ. Management of small corneal infiltrates in contact lens wearers. *Arch Ophthalmol.* 2000;118(2):276–277.
5. Holden BA, Reddy MK, Sankaridurg PR, et al. Contact lens–induced peripheral ulcers with extended wear of disposable hydrogel lenses: Histopathologic observations on the nature and type of corneal infiltrate. *Cornea.* 1999;18(5):538–543.
6. Grant T, Chong MS, Vajdic C, et al. Contact lens induced peripheral ulcers during hydrogel contact lens wear. *CLAO J.* 1998; 24(3):145–151.
7. Snyder C. Infiltrative keratitis with contact lens wear—A review. *J Am Optom Assoc.* 1995;66(3):160–177.
8. Stein RM, Clinch TE, Cohen EJ, et al. Infected vs. sterile corneal infiltrates in contact lens wearers. *Am J Ophthalmol.* 1988; 105(6):632–636.

Pain and Redness with Soft Lens Wear

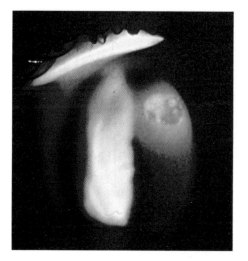

Figure 3-11

History

A 22-year-old Caucasian female presents with a red, painful right eye of 3 days duration. She also reports mucous discharge and photophobia. She states that she is a soft contact lens (CL) wearer who wears her lenses 12–14 hours per day, with occasional overnight wear. She has conventional daily-wear lenses and uses ReNu multipurpose solution. Her current lenses are 6 months old. On further questioning, she reports that she recently went camping and swam in a lake with her lenses on. Her symptoms began the next day. She denies any other ocular or medical history.

Symptoms

- Redness
- Pain
- Mucous discharge
- Photophobia

Clinical Data

- Visual acuity with spectacles:
  OD 20/40 PH-NI
  OS 20/20
- CL prescription: Cibasoft,
  OD 8.6 / 13.8 / –2.00.
  OS 8.6 / 13.8 / –2.50
- Subjective refraction:
  OD –2.00 sphere, 20/40
  OS –2.25 –0.50 × 180, 20/20
- Biomicroscopy: Grade 2 diffuse bulbar injection OD; lid edema and erythema OD; mucopurulent discharge in tear film OD; positively staining white, cloudy lesion 1–2 mm in diameter at 10 o'clock in the corneal mid-periphery, epithelial and anterior stromal, with surrounding haze OD (see Figure 3-11); grade 1 cells in anterior chamber; all structures clear OS

Develop your list of differential diagnoses. Then, based on the clinical data, determine your final diagnosis. Based on your diagnosis, develop your treatment plan.

Differential Diagnoses

- Microbial corneal ulcer
- Infiltrative keratitis
- Pterygium
- Phlyctenule
- Vascularized limbal keratitis

Diagnosis

Microbial corneal ulcer

Management

Contact lens wear was discontinued. The patient was prescribed Ocuflox every 30 minutes for the first 6 hours, then every hour for the remainder of the first day. She was reexamined in 24 hours. The ulcer appeared unchanged, so the treatment was continued. The next day, the ulcer appeared slightly improved, as did the patient's symptoms. The treatment was continued for another day. The following day, the patient seemed more comfortable and the ulcer had begun to heal. The dosage was reduced to every 2 hours. The following day, the ulcer appeared to be healing further so the treatment was maintained. The next day, only a small epithelial defect remained, although the infiltrate and edema were still present. The dosage was reduced to every 4 hours. Two days later, the epithelium still had a small defect but appeared to be healing further. The dosage was further reduced to qid. Three days later, the epithelium showed only negative staining, although the infiltrate was still present. The Ocuflox was maintained at qid. Three days later, the epithelium was healed, with only the infiltrate remaining. The Ocuflox was discontinued. The patient was monitored for another 2 weeks. It was recommended that she not wear contact lenses for approximately 1 month to allow the cornea to heal further. At that time, the patient was refit to a 2-week disposable contact lens to be cleaned and disinfected with QuickCare. The patient gradually built up her wear time and demonstrated no adverse responses at her 1-week, 1-month, and 3-month follow-up visits.

Discussion

Microbial ulcers are the most severe of the contact lens–related complications, yet they occur periodically, especially in extended-wear patients.[1-4] They are characterized by significant symptoms, including intense bulbar redness, photophobia, mucous discharge, and pain.[5-7] These symptoms are the result of the inflammatory response, which is trying aggressively to eliminate the pathogens.[8] Treatment of the ulcer must include antibiotics to kill the microbes and palliative measures to make the patient more comfortable.

Diagnosis of microbial ulcers is not always straightforward.[7,8] Often, infectious ulcers appear very similar to noninfectious ulcers in the early stages. It may not be until several days later that the patient develops more severe symptoms. A history is important in the diagnosis. This patient reported swimming with her lenses on, which makes a microbial etiology more likely. Other positive history elements may include trauma,[5,6,9] chronic overnight wear,[5,6,9–12] lens spoliation,[5,6,10,12] and steroid use.[5,6]

Long-term soft lens wear with conventional daily-wear lenses causes alterations in corneal integrity and metabolism.[10] Predisposing factors include edema, loss of epithelial cells, and abnormal epithelial cell mitosis. These compromises predispose the patient to complications such as corneal ulcers. Regular follow-up visits should include careful evaluation of the cornea with high magnification biomicroscopy with and without fluorescein stain. Any abnormality, including punctate erosions, neovascularization, and microcysts, should be considered signs of corneal distress and addressed by refitting into higher-Dk materials and reducing wear time.

Prior to any treatment, a culture should be taken at the ulcer site. This will aid in tailoring therapeutic treatment to the specific organism involved. Until the culture results arrive, aggressive broad-spectrum therapeutic management should be initiated.[5,9,13] The current standard of care consists of a topical fluoroquinolone or fortified aminoglycosides. Because it is easier to obtain, the fluoroquinolone is usually the drug of choice.[5,9,14] Either ciprofloxacin or ofloxacin should be started immediately. Ciprofloxacin is used q15min for the first 6 hours, then q30min for the remainder of the first day, then qh on the second day. Ofloxacin is used q30min for 6 hours, then qh for the remainder of the first day. Ciprofloxacin ointment is available for use at bedtime if drops cannot be instilled around the clock. The patient should be reexamined the next day. Overnight improvement is unlikely, but the ulcer should look no worse than at initial presentation. Until improvement is noted, the topical fluoroquinolones should be continued qh. The patient should be reexamined each day until improvement is noted. Once the ulcer begins to heal, the dosage can be reduced to q2h, then qid. Ciprofloxacin ointment should be continued at bedtime.

If the lesion fails to improve after the culture results return or if it worsens, medical management must be modified toward the specific organism cultured. If the culture is negative for any organism, more aggressive treatment, such as fortified aminoglycosides, vancomycin, or other penicillin analog, should be instituted. Other organisms, such as protozoa, should be suspected as well. Should treatment fail to improve the ulcer, referral to a corneal specialist may be necessary.

Clinical Pearls

- Infectious ulcers may appear noninfectious in the early stages.
- Infectious ulcers are characterized by severe symptoms and signs.

- Treatment of infectious ulcers should be aggressive.
- Culturing of suspected infectious ulcers is important in managing nonhealing cases.

References

1. Poggio EC, Glynn RJ, Schein OD, et al. The incidence of ulcerative keratitis among users of daily-wear and extended-wear soft contact lenses. *N Engl J Med.* 1989;321(12):779–783.
2. Schein OD, Glynn RJ, Poggio EC, et al. The relative risk of ulcerative keratitis among users of daily-wear and extended-wear soft contact lenses. *N Engl J Med.* 1989;321(12):773–778.
3. Cohen EJ, Fulton JC, Hoffman CJ, et al. Trends in contact lens–associated corneal ulcers. *Cornea.* 1996;15(6):566–570.
4. Liesegang TJ. Contact lens–related microbial keratitis: Part I: Epidemiology. *Cornea.* 1997;16(2):125–131.
5. Stonecipher KG, Jensen H. Diagnosis, laboratory analysis, and treatment of bacterial corneal ulcers. *Optom Clin.* 1995; 4(3):53–64.
6. Silbert JA. Contact lens–induced microbial infections. *Practical Optom.* 1994;5(3):99–104, 128.
7. Stein RM, Clinch TE, Cohen EJ, et al. Infected vs. sterile corneal infiltrates in contact lens wearers. *Am J Ophthalmol.* 1988; 105(6):632–636.
8. Cohen EJ. Management of small corneal infiltrates in contact lens wearers. *Arch Ophthalmol.* 2000;118(2):276–277.
9. Stern GA. Contact lens–associated bacterial keratitis: Past, present, and future. *CLAO J.* 1998;24(1):52–56.
10. Liesegang TJ. Contact lens–related microbial keratitis: Part II: Pathophysiology. *Cornea.* 1997;16(3):265–273.
11. Schein OD, Buehler PO, Stamler JF, et al. The impact of overnight wear on the risk of contact lens–associated ulcerative keratitis. *Arch Ophthalmol.* 1994;112(2):186–190.
12. Laibson PR, Cohen EJ, Rajpal RK. Corneal ulcers related to contact lenses. *CLAO J.* 1993;19(1):73–77.
13. Bennett HGB, Hay J, Kirkness CM, et al. Antimicrobial management of presumed microbial keratitis: Guidelines for treatment of central and peripheral ulcers. *Br J Ophthalmol.* 1998;82(2):137–145.
14. Prajna NV, George C, Selvaraj S, et al. Bacteriologic and clinical efficacy of Ofloxacin 0.3% versus Ciprofloxacin 0.3% ophthalmic solutions in the treatment of patients with culture-positive bacterial keratitis. *Cornea.* 2001;20(2):175–178.

Rigid Gas-Permeable Lens Discomfort

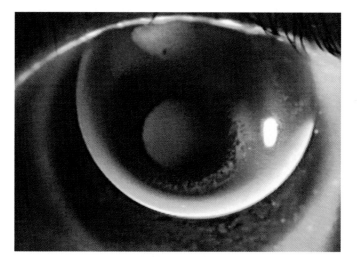

Figure 3-12

History

Patient BB is a 48-year-old Caucasian male who presents for a routine eye examination. He reports that he has been a rigid gas-permeable (RGP) contact lens (CL) wearer for 10 years. His current lenses are 3 years old, and he feels he needs to order a new pair. He has no visual complaints, but his lenses have become less comfortable over the past 3 months. He wears his lenses 18 hours per day, 7 days a week. He uses the Boston Original Care System. He reports no other ocular problems. His ocular history is significant for myopia, astigmatism, and long-standing floaters. His medical history is unremarkable. He takes no medications and has no allergies.

Symptoms

Decreased lens comfort for the past 3 months

Clinical Data

- Visual acuity with CL:
  OD 20/25
  OS 20/30
- Current CL prescription: OU 8.30 / –8.25 / 10.0 / unknown material
- Over-refraction:
  OD –0.50 sphere, 20/20
  OS –0.25 sphere, 20/20
- Lens fit assessment:
  OD extreme superior-central position, no movement on blink, irregular fluorescein pattern with moderate edge lift, thick mucous trapped behind lens (see Figure 3-12)
  OS superior-central position, 2 mm movement on blink, mild apical clearance with mid-peripheral bearing and moderate edge lift
- Keratometry (after lens removal):
  OD 41.75 / 42.50 @ 075, grade 2 distortion
  OS 41.50 / 41.37 @ 090, clear mires
- Corneal topography:
  OD irregular pattern with flat superior-temporal zone and inferior steepening
  OS spherical pattern centrally with small inferior steep zone
- Subjective refraction:
  OD –10.25 –1.00 × 180, 20/20
  OS –10.00 –0.50 × 180, 20/30
- Biomicroscopy:
  OD inferior epithelial staining, RGP imprint, diffuse central SPK
  OS all structures appear clear and healthy

Develop your list of differential diagnoses. Then, based on the clinical data, determine your final diagnosis. Based on your diagnosis, develop your treatment plan.

Differential Diagnoses

- Lens surface deposits
- Corneal abrasion

- RGP adhesion
- Solution preservative allergy

Diagnosis

You determine the patient has RGP adhesion.

Management

RGP lens wear was discontinued OD until corneal topography returned to normal. Because of the patient's high prescription and lack of current spectacles, he was given an Acuvue 8.8 / –9.50 / 14.0 as a temporary lens until the cornea stabilized. He continued to wear his RGP in the left eye. The patient was given nonpreserved artificial tears qid. He was seen over the next 2 weeks for serial topographies, which by then had returned to normal. The patient was then refitted with a more centrally fitting RGP lens. The diameter was reduced, the base curve steepened, and the edge lift decreased: Boston EO / 8.10 / –8.75 / 9.2. This resulted in a slight superior-central lens position and better movement on blink. The patient was also reeducated on proper lens care and the use of rewetting drops.

Discussion

RGP lens adhesion is a relatively common problem,[1] usually multifactorial in etiology. The primary cause is poor lens alignment with the cornea, resulting in areas of touch and vaulting. In most cases, the lens is decentered past the limbus,[2] creating a steep fit over the flat portion of the cornea. Low axial edge lift is commonly present. This creates lens flexure and suction that causes the lens to stick to the cornea.[2,3] Additionally, a thin postlens tear layer increases the chance that the lens will adhere to the eye. As aqueous fluid is pushed out from under the lens, a more viscous mucoid layer remains behind, acting as a glue to adhere the lens to the cornea.[4,5] A thicker, more stable tear film provides a cushion on which the lens can glide with each blink, minimizing the chance that the lens will adhere. A dirty lens surface also contributes to the problem by attracting mucous to the post-lens space. Adhesion is more likely with extended-wear RGP lenses.[1–6]

RGP adhesion is very simple to diagnose. The lens is stuck to the cornea, and it takes a moderate amount of manipulation to free the lens. Again, the lens is almost always decentered past the limbus, and mucous is present behind the lens. Corneal staining is present adjacent to the lens edge, due to drying of the tear film. On removal, a lens imprint is visible, and more corneal staining is present where the lens is adherent.

Because the lens is decentered and pressing into the cornea, corneal distortion always results. The irregularity is asymmetric, with the area under the lens becoming flat and the area outside the lens becoming steep. If the lens decenters superiorly, as often occurs in an extreme lid-attached fit, the resulting topography mimics a keratoconus pattern, often referred to as *pseudokeratoconus*.[7-9] This distortion also is present on keratometry, although the pseudokeratoconus pattern is not evident. Topography is the most important objective measure in monitoring resolution of the corneal distortion. In many cases, subjective refraction shows irregular astigmatism and reduced best-corrected visual acuity. As the topography normalizes, the refraction returns to normal with good acuity.

Management of the patient can be quite difficult. First, studies investigating parameter changes to alleviate lens adhesion are sparse, and those that have been done find somewhat contradictory results.[1,6,10] In addition, because the patient is usually relatively asymptomatic,[1] he or she must be made to understand why it is important to discontinue lens wear. Showing the patient the irregular topography and videotaping or photographing the adherent lens can be valuable in explaining the situation. When the topography is normalized, it is important to perform a careful refit to prevent recurrence of the problem.

The first step is to try on the patient's old lenses to visualize the fitting relationship. If the lens decenters, the goal is to fit a lens that centers. If the lens is not a lid-attachment fit, increasing lens diameter to improve centration is a good first step. The base curve should be optimized as well, to provide moderate edge lift. If the edge lift appears too high or too wide, the peripheral curves must be steepened to improve centration.

If the old lens lid attaches, then the diameter should be decreased to allow better lens centration. The final base curve is usually steeper and should allow apical alignment or slight clearance to ensure that the lens will not decenter. The periphery should be optimized to allow moderate edge lift. These fine-tuning adjustments help decrease the chance of adhesion.[10]

After refitting, lens wear should be accompanied by rewetting drops, especially in patients with suboptimal tear films.[6] Proper lens care with an abrasive daily cleaner and enzymatic cleaning should be reemphasized. Finally, annual exams and lens replacements[6] when necessary should be recommended to prevent recurrent lens adhesion.

Clinical Pearls

- RGP lens adhesion is characterized by an immobile lens, post-lens mucous, corneal staining, and corneal distortion.
- RGP lens adhesion occurs more frequently with decentered lenses and extended wear.
- Patients with corneal distortion must be monitored until the corneal topography and refraction are stable.
- RGP refitting should emphasize a central lens position, apical alignment fluorescein pattern, and moderate edge lift.

References

1. Kenyon E, Polse KA, Mandell RB. Rigid contact lens adherence: Incidence, severity and recovery. *J Am Optom Assoc.* 1988; 59(3):167–174.
2. Swarbrick HA, Holden BA. Rigid gas-permeable lens binding: Significance and contributing factors. *Am J Optom Physiol Optics.* 1987;64(11):815–823.
3. Goldberg JB. RGP contact lens adherence: Flexure or tear film thinning—Can we define the cause? *Int Contact Lens Clin.* 1994;21(1):26–28.
4. Swarbrick HA, Holden BA. Ocular characteristics associated with rigid gas-permeable lens adherence. *Optom Vis Sci.* 1996;73(7):473–481.
5. Taylor AJ, Wilson SDR. Post-lens tear film thinning in rigid gas-permeable lenses. *Optom Vis Sci.* 1995;72(12):849–856.
6. Woods CA, Efron N. Regular replacement of rigid contact lenses alleviates binding to the cornea. *Int Contact Lens Clin.* 1996;23(1):13–18.
7. Shovlin JP, DePaolis MD, Kame RT. Contact lens–induced corneal warpage syndrome vs. keratoconus. *Contact Lens Forum.* 1986;11(8):32–36.
8. Lebow KA, Grohe RM. Differentiating contact lens–induced warpage from true keratoconus using corneal topography. *CLAO J.* 1999;25(2):114–122.
9. Eghbali F. Keratoconus suspect or pseudokeratoconus? *Contact Lens Spectrum.* 1997;12(12):30–32.

10. Swarbrick HA, Holden BA. Effects of lens parameter variation on rigid gas-permeable lens adherence. *Optom Vis Sci.* 1996;73(3):144–155.

Painful Red Eye with Soft Lens Wear

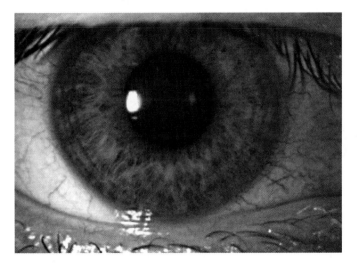

Figure 3-13

History

A 29-year-old Caucasian female presents with a painful red eye on awakening this morning. She also reports severe photophobia and worsening of symptoms after she removes her lenses. She currently wears extended-wear soft lenses, routinely for up to 14 continuous days. Her current lenses are 7 months old. She uses Bausch & Lomb saline and an enzymatic cleaner to clean and enzyme the lenses when she removes them. Her left eye is fine. She denies any ocular or systemic health problems. She takes oral contraceptives and has no allergies.

Symptoms

- Redness
- Severe pain
- Severe photophobia
- Symptoms on awakening, worse after lens removal

Clinical Data

- Visual acuity with spectacles:
  OD 20/80 PH-NI
  OS 20/20
- External examination:
  OD Grade 3 bulbar injection (see Figure 3-13), profuse tearing
  OS Clear
- Biomicroscopy (after instillation of 1 gtt 0.5% proparacaine):
  OD Several fine corneal infiltrates, grade 1 diffuse punctate erosions, grade 2 stromal edema
  OS Grade 2 microcysts, trace diffuse punctate erosions
- CL specifications: B&L U4,
  OD –6.00
  OS –4.75
- Lens examination: Both lenses appear mildly protein coated, lens case is dirty

  Develop your list of differential diagnoses. Then, based on the clinical data, determine your final diagnosis. Based on your diagnosis, develop your treatment plan.

Differential Diagnoses

- Corneal ulcer
- Contact lens acute red eye
- Soft lens–associated corneal hypoxia
- Viral conjunctivitis
- Bacterial conjunctivitis
- Recurrent corneal erosion

Diagnosis

Contact lens acute red eye (CLARE)

Management

The patient was prescribed Polytrim drops qid and scheduled for a follow-up visit in 24 hours. The next day, her symptoms were much reduced, though the infiltrates were still present. She was instructed to continue the Polytrim drops and return in 3 days. At this visit, she reported that her symptoms had resolved and that she was eager to start lens wear. She was advised not to wear her lenses until the infiltrates resolved and then limit lenses to daily wear. Two weeks later, she was refitted with a higher-water-content disposable lens to increase oxygen transmissibility and ensure that she wears clean lenses. She remained asymptomatic at her 1- and 3-month progress evaluations and reported that she adheres to the daily-wear schedule.

Discussion

The presence of fine infiltrates should make one suspect corneal infection. The rapid and severe unilateral presentation seen in this case is not consistent with viral or bacterial conjunctivitis. Although hyperacute conjunctivitis can present this way, it usually has significant mucous discharge, which is absent in this case. Recurrent corneal erosions can be painful and often occur on awakening, but the pain tends to decrease over time. Soft lens–associated corneal hypoxia (SLACH) is similar to this case but would present with a relatively large corneal epithelial defect, which is absent here.

This patient's symptoms are typical for contact lens acute red eye (CLARE). Symptoms appear immediately on awakening after overnight soft lens wear, sometimes waking the patient due to the severe pain.[1-4] Long-term soft lens extended wear compromises corneal integrity and function such that it is susceptible to acute inflammatory responses. It is thought that gram-positive[2,5-7] or gram-negative[2,3,8] bacteria or their toxins may become trapped under a tight-fitting soft lens, triggering the inflammatory response. The resulting pain and photophobia increase on lens removal because of exposure of the compromised cornea and the return of corneal sensitivity that had decreased due to extended wear.

Treatment of CLARE must address the patient's symptoms as well as management of lens wearing and care habits. A broad-spectrum antibiotic, such as a fluoroquinolone or aminoglycoside, should be instituted qid for the first 24–48 hours,[3] although CLARE has been shown that to resolve without antibiotic treatment.[2] A frank infection usually is not present, although a compromised epithelium puts the patient at risk. Extended wear alters the ocular flora such that virulent gram-negative bacteria, such as *Pseudomonas aeruginosa*, are present[9] and more adherent to the corneal epithelium.[10] Therefore, the antibiotic must have good gram-negative activity. A cycloplegic decreases photophobia by relaxing the ciliary body, and an oral analgesic can deaden some of the pain for the first day.

On resolution, the patient should be reeducated on his or her wearing schedule. Extended wear should be terminated, and patients often resume daily wear with the same lens type. If the patient is wearing a tight, low-Dk lens, a looser, higher-Dk brand should be refit. A silicone hydrogel may be a good solution if it demonstrates adequate movement. Proper lens care and case maintenance are important as well. Use of saline and enzymatic cleaners alone is insufficient for proper disinfection. A proper care system with sufficient action against gram-negative bacteria should be prescribed. These measures help prevent a recurrence of CLARE.

Clinical Pearls

- CLARE is caused by chronic soft lens extended wear and the presence of bacteria, particularly gram-negative species.
- CLARE is noninfectious but predisposes the patient to secondary infection.
- Broad-spectrum antibiotics, cycloplegics, and oral analgesics are used to treat CLARE.
- Refitting and reeducation are key to preventing recurrence.

References

1. Zantos SG, Holden BA. Ocular changes associated with continuous wear of contact lenses. *Aust J Optom*. 1978;61:418–426.
2. Holden BA, Sankaridurg PR, Jalbert I. Adverse events and infection: Which ones and how many? In: Sweeney DF (ed). *Silicone Hydrogels—The Rebirth of Continuous Wear Contact Lenses*. Oxford: Butterworth–Heinemann, 2000:168–175.
3. Silbert JA. Inflammatory responses in contact lens wear. In: Silbert JA (ed). *Anterior Segment Complications of Contact Lens Wear*, 2nd ed. Boston: Butterworth–Heinemann, 2000:125–126.
4. Millis E. Contact lenses and the red eye. *Contact Lens Anterior Eye* (suppl). 1997;20(2):S5–S10.

5. Swarbrick HA, Holden BA. Complications of hydrogel extended-wear lenses. In: Silbert JA (ed). *Anterior Segment Complications of Contact Lens Wear*, 2nd ed. Boston: Butterworth–Heinemann, 2000:295–296.

6. Wu PZJ, Thakur A, Stapleton F, Willcox MDP. Staphylococcus aureus causes acute inflammatory episodes in the cornea during contact lens wear. *Clin Exper Ophthalmol.* 2000;28:194–196.

7. Sankaridurg PR, Sharma S, Willcox M, et al. Colonization of hydrogel lenses with *Streptococcus pneumoniae*: Risk of development of corneal infiltrates. *Cornea.* 1999;18(3):289–295.

8. Holden BA, LaHood D, Grant T, et al. Gram-negative bacteria can induce contact lens–related acute red eye (CLARE) responses. *CLAO J.* 1996;22(1):47–52.

9. Stapleton F, Willcox MDP, Fleming CM, et al. Changes in the ocular biota with time in extended-wear and daily-wear disposable contact lens use. *Infect Immun.* 1995;63(11):4501–4505.

10. Fleiszig SM, Efron N, Pier GB. Extended contact lens wear enhances *Pseudomonas aeruginosa* adherence to human corneal epithelium. *Invest Ophthalmol Vis Sci.* 1992;33(10):2908–2916.

PART 4

Specialty Contact Lens Fitting Dilemmas

CASE 4-1

Uncomfortable Rigid Gas-Permeable Lens in Keratoconus
Edward S. Bennett

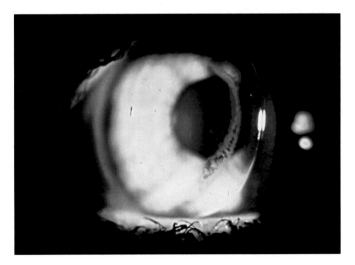

Figure 4-1

History

Patient CG is a 42-year-old female who first presented to the University of Missouri-St. Louis School of Optometry in March 1993. She had been diagnosed with keratoconus in 1978. She was fit into a PMMA lens (soon to be refit into a rigid gas-permeable [RGP] lens) in the right eye and a soft contact lens (SCL) for the left eye. I received a call from a local optometrist who wanted to refer her to my care. She had been severely limiting the wearing time (approximately 5 hours) in the more advanced right eye due to dryness and accompanying lens awareness. Her optometrist attempted numerous RGP contact lens (CL) designs on that eye with little success. As a result of the moderate severity of

173

the keratoconus in that eye combined with her limited wearing time, he often recommended referral for a penetrating keratoplasty. In fact, at the time of her first visit to our clinic, she had an appointment scheduled with a corneal surgeon for a consultation.

Symptoms

- Limited wearing time with RGP contact lens OD
- Lens dryness OD
- Lens awareness OD

Clinical Data

- Entering visual acuity:
  OD (with RGP) 20/30[+2]
  OS (with SCL) 20/25
- Lens specifications:
  OD 6.52 / –8.50 / 7.6 / 6.0 / 0.14
  OS Unknown soft lens material / –2.00D
- Contact lens evaluation:
  OD Good centration, less than 1 mm lag with the blink; alignment to slight touch centrally; very little peripheral clearance with fluorescein application (see Figure 4-1)
  OS Good movement and centration but soft lens was heavily deposited
- Biomicroscopy:
  OD Dense central scar, Fleischer ring, and numerous Vogt's straie; mild coalescence of central staining
  OS All structures appear clear and healthy
- Tear break-up time: 5 seconds OU
- Pachometry: OD 0.442 mm
- Keratometry: EyeSys,
  OD 54.62 / 55.37
  OS 43.25 @ 175; 43.75 @ 085
- Manifest refraction:
  OD Difficult to obtain
  OS –2.25 –0.25 × 145

Differential Diagnoses

- Unilateral keratoconus
- Lens adherence
- Flat-fitting lens

- Steep-fitting lens
- Steep peripheral curves

Diagnosis

Lens adherence in a unilateral keratoconus patient due to steep peripheral curves

Management

The right eye was refit with a different RGP design, and the left eye was refit into an RGP to improve vision and maintain the same modality for both eyes. Several lenses were attempted on the right eye prior to a successful fit. Ultimately, she ended up with this lens with a three-point touch-fitting relationship:

OD FluoroPerm 30 / 6.89 / –5.75 / 8.8 / 7.6 / 7.8 @ 0.3 / 9.8 @ 0.3 / 0.15

The left eye achieved an alignment fitting relationship with the following lens:

OS Fluoroperm 30 / 7.85 / –2.00 / 8.8 / 7.6 / 8.8 @ 0.3 / 10.8 @ 0.3 / 0.20
Visual acuity (with lenses): OD $20/25^{-2}$; OS $20/25^{+2}$

CG was able to attain 14 hours of wear with these lenses and was evaluated several times between April 1993 and October 1994. On each visit, it was noted that lens movement was insufficient (<1 mm) for the right lens, and intermittent adherence was often noted as well. She experienced coalesced central corneal staining and, on one occasion (August 1993), a mild corneal abrasion. At the October 1994 visit, it was recommended that she return in 1 month for a follow-up evaluation and probable refit of the right lens. However, she was not evaluated again until June 1995. Based on the absence of lens movement with the blink at this visit and the mild discomfort she was experiencing with lens wear, it was decided to refit her with another design. It was noted that she had moderate central bearing and peripheral seal off with lens wear and central coalesced staining after lens removal.

She was refit into the Rose-K lens (Lens Dynamics) for keratoconus with the following parameters:

OD Fluoroperm 30 / 6.60 / –7.50 / 8.7 / 6.6 / high edge lift

The high edge lift was selected to increase peripheral clearance, and ideally, the small optical zone diameter will be beneficial in enhancing lens movement with the blink.

On dispensing the new lens, her visual acuity was 20/20^{-1} OD. A three-point touch-fitting relationship was present with adequate peripheral clearance. CG was satisfied with the comfort and vision of this lens. She followed up five times between October 1995 and August 1996; the latter represented her last visit at the clinic, as she was moving to California. At her last visit, her visual acuity was 20/25 with very mild central pooling and adequate peripheral clearance with fluorescein. Between 1 and 2 mm lens lag was present with the blink, and the lens was well-centered. There were no signs of adherence and only minimal corneal staining; the patient was very satisfied with the comfort and vision of this lens. She wears her lenses 14 hours a day, and her refraction and simulated keratometry readings (EyeSys) are

OD –9.75 –2.50 × 050, 20/40
OD 52.89 @ 138; 50.29 @ 048

Discussion

Lens adherence with a rigid lens is not difficult to diagnose. In the case of CG, it is apparent that some clinical signs of intermittent adherence were evident prior to the lens becoming constantly adherent. These clinical signs included limited lens movement, mild adherence ring on lens removal, and corneal staining resulting from trapped debris. As it is possible that the patient may not be symptomatic, a thorough slit-lamp examination—both with and without lens wear—is important. As adherence can be caused by a nonalignment fluorescein pattern as well as by peripheral seal off, it is a condition that often occurs with an RGP fit in keratoconus. Diffuse or coalesced corneal staining, so common in keratoconus, in many cases may be caused by trapped debris from a constantly or intermittently adherent rigid lens.

The etiology of lens-to-cornea adherence is controversial.[1,2] However, with the less than alignment-fitting relationship apparent with a spherical lens on an irregular cornea and the variable size and location of the affected region of the cornea, it makes sense that adherence is more likely to occur with these patients than with individuals having regular corneas. To minimize peripheral seal off, the use of a flat, wide peripheral curve has been recommended.[3] Likewise, reducing the optical zone as the base curve steepens typically results in better centration and better lens-to-cornea alignment. In fact, it is not uncommon to have an optical zone value similar to the base curve radius in millimeters.

In this particular case, the patient had numerous failures with RGP lens wear prior to visiting the clinic. The first lenses attempted had a relatively large optical zone diameter and a conventional peripheral curve radius and width. Over time this contributed to intermittent and finally constant adherence of lens to cornea. She was refit with the Rose-K lens design, which is based on a complex mathematical computer model that yields thousands of peripheral curve combinations.[4] It customarily has a small optical zone and five to six blended peripheral curve radii. It can be ordered in a low, standard, and high edge lift; the flat or high edge lift is 1 mm flatter than the standard edge lift. The use of this edge lift, in combination with the small optical zone used in the Rose-K design, resulted in good centration and lens movement with the blink, adequate peripheral clearance, minimal corneal staining, and very good patient satisfaction.

Clinical Pearls

- RGP lens adherence is more likely to occur with irregular cornea patients, due to a less than alignment fitting relationship and the variable size and location of the affected region of the cornea.
- To minimize peripheral seal off, use a flat, wide peripheral curve and reduce the optical zone as the base curve steepens.
- In keratoconus, it is not uncommon to have an optical zone value similar to the base curve radius in millimeters.

References

1. Swarbrick HA, Holden BA. Rigid gas-permeable lens binding: Significance and contributing factors. *Am J Optom Physiol Opt.* 1987;64(11):815–823.
2. Bennett ES, Grohe RM. How to solve stuck lens syndrome. *Rev Optom.* 1987;124(12):51–52.
3. Bennett ES. A commonsense approach to fitting keratoconus with RGP lenses. *Optom Today.* 1997;5(2):25–27.
4. Caroline PJ, Norman C, Andre M. The latest lens design for keratoconus. *Contact Lens Spectrum.* 1997;12(8):36–41.

Bifocal Contact Lens Problem

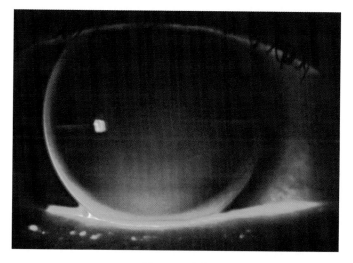

Figure 4-2

History

Patient CF, a 52-year-old Caucasian female, presents for her annual eye examination inquiring about bifocal contact lenses. With her current soft contact lenses (CL), she complains of poor distance vision, especially at night, and decreasing near vision. Her last pair of soft lenses was slightly undercorrected to help her at near. She also reports that she has dynamic visual demands on the job, where she must view distance, intermediate, and near objects in rapid sequence. Her current lenses allow her to perform these visual tasks with great difficulty. She wears her lenses 15 hours a day. She uses a generic multipurpose solution to clean and disinfect her lenses daily and enzymes her lenses once a week. Her ocular and medical histories are unremarkable. She takes no medications and reports no known allergies.

Symptoms

Poor near and intermediate vision with her current contact lenses

Clinical Data

- Entering visual acuity at distance with CL:
  OD 20/50
  OS 20/50
- Over-refraction:
  OD –1.00 –0.50 × 030, 20/20–
  OS –0.75 –0.50 × 170, 20/20–
- Entering VA at near with CL:
  OD 20/40
  OS 20/60
- Contact lens parameters:
  OD CSI Clarity / 8.6 / 13.8 / –2.50
  OS Cibasoft / 8.6 / 13.8 / –3.50
- Fit assessment: OU centered, 0.25 mm movement on blink, moderate protein film
- Keratometry:
  OD 40.50 / 41.12 @ 090
  OS 40.87 / 41.12 @ 090
- Subjective refraction:
  OD –3.50 –0.50 × 030, 20/20
  OS –3.75 –0.50 × 170, 20/20
  Add +2.00
- External exam: All structures appear clear and quiet OU; palpebral fissure 8 mm OD and 9 mm OS; lower eyelid 1 mm above limbus OD and tangent to limbus OS; pupil diameter 5 mm in dark and 2.5 mm in light OU
- Biomicroscopy: All structures appear clear and quiet OU

Based on the clinical data presented, determine a list of contact lens fitting options. Then, determine the most appropriate option and the initial prescription.

Fitting Options

- Spherical soft lens update
- Rigid gas-permeable (RGP) lenses
- Monovision
- Multifocals

Management

Several options were presented to the patient, including monovision, soft multifocals, and rigid multifocals. Initially, the patient rejected the idea of rigid lenses, based on a prior bad experience with PMMA lenses. She also rejected monovision because she would lose her binocularity. The patient was then diagnostically fit with a center-near aspheric soft multifocal and later with a distance-center aspheric RGP multifocal but was unable to achieve clarity at near with either option. After more discussion and reassurance, she was refit with a translating RGP bifocal design: Solitaire II / Fluoro-Perm 60,

8.33 / –2.25 / +2.00 add / 9.4 × 9.0 / 7.8 / 4.0 seg ht / 2.25 pd BD
8.33 / –2.50 / +2.00 add / 9.4 × 9.0 / 7.8 / 4.0 seg ht / 2.25 pd BD

These lenses yielded distance VA of OD 20/25 and OS 20/20– and near VA of 20/20 OU. The lenses positioned on the lower lids with good movement and rapid return after blink. Both lenses fit with apical alignment and moderate peripheral clearance. The segment line was horizontal with good rotational stability. The lenses demonstrated good translation on down gaze. The patient noted occasional blurry distance vision and blurry intermediate vision. The segment line OD was found to be too high, bisecting the pupil (see Figure 4-2). The right lens was then truncated another 0.3 mm, and the segment line took on a more acceptable position.

On follow-up, the patient still noticed blur in the intermediate range but good distance and near vision. A trifocal design with a progressive intermediate range was ordered to try to provide intermediate-range clarity. After 2 weeks of trial with this design, the patient was unable to adapt to the small intermediate zone. She found that her vision was more variable, and she could not appreciate clarity at intermediate distances.

She was then refit with Solitaire II bifocal lenses with unequal add powers. Because she is left eye dominant, the add power of her left lens was decreased to +1.00, providing her with distance vision in both eyes, intermediate vision in her left eye, and near vision in her right eye. With this combination, she was able to view all distances comfortably. Her final contact lens prescription is:

- Tru-form Optics Solitaire II,
  OD 8.33 / –2.25 / +2.00 add / 9.4 × 8.7 / 3.7 seg ht / 2.25 pd BD
  OS 8.33 / –2.50 / +1.00 add / 9.4 × 9.0 / 4.0 seg ht / 2.25 pd BD

- Distance VA:
  - OD 20/20
  - OS 20/20
- Near VA:
  - OD 20/20
  - OS 20/25

Discussion

This patient had a complex fit for several reasons. First, she had high expectations for clear vision. Second, she had a relatively high add requirement. Third, she had to switch fixation rapidly while on the job. Finally, she had a previous bad experience with hard lenses that had to be overcome. Although it took several tries to find a good option for this patient, in the end, she found a satisfactory option.

It is well known that RGP lenses provide clearer vision than soft lenses.[1-5] This is particularly true in cases of corneal astigmatism and when trying to fit multifocal contact lenses with high add powers. Multifocal soft lenses do not deliver consistent visual results, especially for a patient with high expectations. However, because of the patient's resistance to rigid lenses, soft lenses had to be tried first. Once she saw that they would not work for her, she was better able to accept the RGP lenses. It would have been much more difficult to get her to accept the RGP lenses without first trying the soft lens options.

Aspheric RGP multifocals provide a clearer alternative to soft multifocals.[1-5] However, they rely on simultaneous vision to some degree, just as soft lenses do. Therefore, the multifocal optics introduce some amount of blur. The advantages of aspheric designs include a full range of vision (distance, intermediate, near) and a concentric add zone (can appreciate near vision in any position of gaze).[1-5] Therefore, if the patient could appreciate vision clear enough for her demands, this lens design would have worked well. However, the patient was unhappy with her near vision with this design.

The alternating RGP bifocal design delivers the visual clarity this patient demands. Although there is a learning curve to using them properly, once the patient becomes accustomed to proper viewing and blinking habits, she will appreciate the best possible multifocal vision of any contact lens. Some fine-tuning of the bifocal contact lens led to improved performance. First, the segment height of the right lens was too high, causing her distance vision to fluctuate during blinks. This can be distracting during highly visual distance tasks, such as driving. It is fairly easy to truncate a lens in-office using a fine-grain file or modification unit. The RGP lab also can truncate the lens. Second, the +2.00 add power was too high for the patient's intermediate vision tasks. By decreasing the add in her dominant eye, she could appreciate clarity at this distance. Even though trifocal or progressive intermediate designs work for some, this patient was unable to use the different zones efficiently and became frustrated with the blurry vision. By limiting the number of zones per lens to two, the learning curve is simpler, and the patient can learn to use the lens more quickly.

This case demonstrates how persistence to a logical progression of options can make even the most demanding patients successful with bifocal contact lenses.

Clinical Pearls

- Presbyopes with moderate astigmatism, high adds, and high expectations are more successful with RGP designs.
- Although aspheric multifocals provide a full range of vision, visual acuity sometimes is compromised.
- Alternating design multifocals can provide intermediate-range vision by decreasing the add in the dominant eye or by using trifocal or progressive intermediate designs.

References

1. Watanabe R. Presbyopia: Contact lenses 2000. *Contact Lens Spectrum*. 2000;15(5):41–47.
2. Edwards K. Contact lens problem-solving: Bifocal contact lenses. *Optician*. 1999;218(5721):26–32.
3. Bennett ES, Schwartz CA. Troubleshooting multifocal RGPs. *Contact Lens Spectrum*. 1998;13(10):49–51.
4. Hansen DW. Rigid bifocal contact lenses. *Optom Clin*. 1994;4(1):103–119.
5. Lebow KA. Contemporary RGP bifocals: Fitting and followup. *Eyequest*. 1992;2(5):34–46.

.

CASE 4-3

Difficult Rigid Gas-Permeable Lens Fit

Timothy B. Edrington

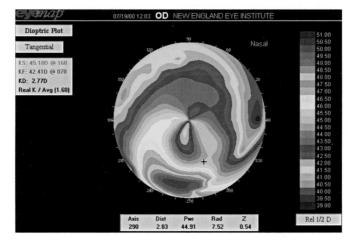

Figure 4-3

History

A 32-year-old male presents with a history of spectacle wear since the age of 17. He had been informed that he had too much astigmatism to successfully wear either soft or rigid contact lenses. One year ago, he was diagnosed as a keratoconus suspect. Rigid gas-permeable (RGP) contact lenses (CL) were prescribed, but lens wear was discontinued after several prescriptions failed to achieve adequate vision and comfort. The remainder of the case history is unremarkable.

Symptoms

- Poor vision and comfort with RGP lenses
- High astigmatism, keratoconus suspect

Clinical Data

- Habitual spectacles and resultant visual acuity:
  OD +1.75 –5.75 × 082, 20/25$^{+3/6}$
  OS +2.00 –6.25 × 097, 20/30$^{+2/6}$
- Simulated keratometry with videokeratography revealed:
  OD 41.46 @ 072 / 46.23 @ 162
  OS 42.77 @ 100 / 51.76 @ 010
- Manifest refraction and resultant visual acuity:
  OD +1.50 –6.00 × 088, 20/20$^{-2/6}$
  OS +2.00 –6.50 × 092, 20/25$^{+2/6}$
- Slit-lamp biomicroscopy: Clear cornea with no Fleischer's ring or Vogt's striae. However, corneal thinning was observed inferiorly in both eyes. Corneal topography showed an area of corneal steepening superior to the inferior limbal thinning, resulting in a teardrop or gull-wing appearance (see Figure 4-3 for corneal topography of a different yet similar case).

Differential Diagnosis[1]

- Keratoconus
- Pellucid marginal degeneration
- Terrien's marginal degeneration
- Mooren's ulcer
- Marginal furrow degeneration

Diagnosis

Pellucid marginal degeneration

Management

Rigid contact lenses were diagnostically fitted, but adequate lens centration was not achieved. All diagnostic lenses positioned extremely inferiorly and were not picked up by the upper eyelid on the blink. A lid-attachment fit was not considered because the patient's upper eyelid position was superior to the limbus.

The patient was empirically prescribed custom soft toric contact lenses. The lens brand and parameters were selected to maximize lens rotational stability. After one lens exchange, the patient was satisfied with his vision, the lens fit was optimal, and the corneal response was satisfactory. On follow-up visits, special attention was given to the cornea's response to the wear of the lenses. This response was monitored by thorough slit-lamp examination, looking for corneal staining, striae, or inferior neovascularization due to the thick lens profile. Videokeratography was performed to evaluate any changes in corneal topography, especially inferiorly, due to localized swelling.

Discussion

Correct diagnosis is critical in properly managing pellucid marginal corneal degeneration. Patients with pellucid marginal degeneration are often misdiagnosed as keratoconic, probably due to the rareness[2] of pellucid and the high degree of corneal toricity and steep keratometry readings. Keratoconus patients generally present with one or more of the following corneal findings: Fleischer's ring, Vogt's striae, or corneal scarring.[1] These slit-lamp findings may be present with pellucid patients, but generally they are absent.[3] Also, the location of the corneal thinning is different. The area of corneal thinning usually is central or slightly inferior for keratoconus, whereas the thinning is adjacent to the inferior limbus for pellucid marginal degeneration.[3] It is common for pellucid marginal degeneration patients to have high amounts of against-the-rule astigmatism,[1,2] whereas the manifest refraction in keratoconus often reveals oblique or irregular astigmatism. The corneal steepening superior to the inferior limbal thinning results in a teardrop or gull-wing appearance of the corneal topography, which is pathognomonic for pellucid marginal degeneration.

Other corneal diseases to rule out are Terrien's marginal degeneration (corneal steepening primarily superior-nasal), Mooren's ulcer (an autoimmune response to a corneal injury), and marginal furrow degeneration (peripheral corneal thinning occurring within the area of corneal arcus, primarily in the elderly).

Pellucid marginal degeneration patients with mild and moderate disease generally have acceptable vision through their manifest refraction.[2] High amounts of against-the-rule astigmatism are common, but the central cornea may have only minimal amounts of distortion. Therefore, spectacles or soft toric contact lenses initially may be good options for vision correction. More advanced patients, with distorted or irregular corneas, benefit from the optics provided by rigid contact lenses. Rigid contact lenses tend to position inferiorly on pellucid corneas;[2,3] therefore, a large overall diameter or a lid-attached fit is necessary for the optic zone to position in front of the pupil. Even though pellucid marginal degeneration patients often have large amounts of against-the-rule corneal toricity, a bitoric design usually is unwarranted. Most of the lens decentration is inferior, not nasal or temporal. Piggybacking a rigid lens on top of a soft lens generally does not adequately assist in lens centration. Options such as soft-rigid hybrids (Soft-Perm), soft lenses with a rigid lens insert (FlexLens), and large overall diameter "rigid" lenses (Macrolens or Epicon) may be prescribed if adequate centration is not achieved with rigid contact lenses and if vision is not acceptable with spectacles or soft toric contact lenses. In severe cases, surgical procedures such as penetrating keratoplasty or lamellar grafting may be indicated.

Clinical Pearls

- Correct diagnosis is critical in properly managing pellucid marginal corneal degeneration patients.
- Pellucid marginal degeneration generally is misdiagnosed as keratoconus.
- Videokeratography is of paramount help in differentially diagnosing the condition and understanding the contour of the cornea to assist the eyecare practitioner in fitting contact lenses.

References

1. Krachmer JH. Pellucid marginal corneal degeneration. *Arch Ophthalmol.* 1978;96(7):1217–1221.
2. Biswas S, Brahma A, Tromans C, Ridgway A. Management of pellucid marginal corneal degeneration. *Eye.* 2000;14(4):629–634.
3. Krachmer JH, Feder RS, Belin MW. Keratoconus and related non-inflammatory corneal thinning disorders. *Surv Ophthalmol.* 1984;28(4):293–322.

CASE 4-4

Postsurgical Glare

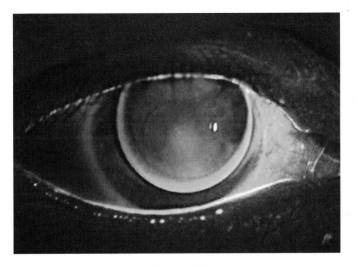

Figure 4-4

History

A 43-year-old Caucasian male presents for a contact lens refitting. He complains of glare and haze, OD more than OS, that worsens at night with his rigid gas-permeable (RGP) contact lenses (CL). He has worn RGP contact lenses for 17 years. He has a history of keratomileusis OD in 1983 that was relatively unsuccessful. Since that time, he has worn a standard RGP lens to correct the residual myopia. His left eye is moderately myopic. His average wear time is 15 hours a day. He uses the Boston Original care system to clean his lenses daily. His ocular history is otherwise unremarkable. His medical history is significant for asthma, for which he uses an albuterol inhaler. He has no known allergies.

Symptoms

Glare with an RGP lens on a post-refractive-surgery cornea

Clinical Data

- VA with CL:
  OD 20/25
  OS 20/25
- Over-refraction:
  OD Plano sphere, 20/25
  OS –0.50 sphere, 20/20–
- RGP contact lens parameters:
  OD 8.20 / –7.00 / 9.6 / unknown design and material
  OS 8.10 / –7.00 / 9.6 / unknown design and material
- Lens fit assessment:
  OD Superior position with lid attachment, minimal movement, apical touch with moderate peripheral clearance (see Figure 4-4)
  OS Superior central position with lid attachment, 2-3 mm movement, apical touch with moderate peripheral clearance
- Biomicroscopy:
  OD Para-central scarring s/p keratomileusis, central cornea clear, all other structures clear and healthy
  OS All structures clear and healthy
- Keratometry:
  OD 39.87 sphere, grade 2 distortion
  OS 41.75 sphere, no distortion
- Subjective refraction:
  OD –6.25 –0.75 × 180, 20/40^{+2}
  OS –9.00 –0.50 × 010, 20/25
- Corneal topography:
  OD Central flat zone with mid-peripheral steepening
  OS Normal with-the-rule bowtie pattern

Based on the clinical data, develop your list of differential diagnoses. Then, determine your final diagnosis and develop your treatment plan.

Differential Diagnoses

- Optic zone too small
- Lens decentration
- Scarring from keratomileusis

Diagnosis

Glare from lens decentration and scarring from keratomileusis

Management

The right eye was refit with a reverse geometry design RGP contact lens to promote centration:

OD Boston EO 8.40 / –6.00 / 10.4 / reverse geometry with 3.00 D steeper secondary curve

With this lens, the patient achieved 20/20– vision with decreased glare. The lens centered well after a blink with mild apical clearance, mid-peripheral alignment, and moderate peripheral clearance. The left lens was unchanged. The patient was educated on the sources of his glare, including the scarring from the keratomileusis surgery.

Discussion

Glare or visual flare is a common complaint following refractive surgery procedures.[1-4] Radial keratotomy, photorefractive keratectomy, and even LASIK produce some amount of glare for most patients. Keratomileusis, one of the precursors to LASIK, is an uncommonly performed surgery that involves removing a button of central cornea with a keratome, freezing and reshaping it with a cryolathe, and suturing it back into place.[1] Historically, it has not been a very successful procedure, and patients are often left with residual myopia and irregular astigmatism. In addition, the junctional area between the host cornea and the reshaped button scars quite extensively, resulting in a ring of scarring surrounding a central clear zone. Patients experience varying amounts of glare depending on the extent of the scarring and the patient's pupil diameter.

The patient's glare is not entirely due to the surgical scarring. Evaluation of the RGP fit reveals a second cause: excessive decentration. The lens positioned superiorly, and as a result, the peripheral curves passed through the pupillary zone and the patient viewed through multiple curves and junctions. This is a problem that may be reduced through careful refitting. However, it may not be completely resolved, due to the difficulty in centering a postsurgical RGP contact lens. In addition, the patient still encounters glare from the surgical scarring even with the most central lens position.

Inspection of the corneal topography reveals a typical post-refractive surgery pattern: a flat central zone surrounded by a steeper mid-peripheral cornea. Parameter changes that help center an RGP lens on this type of topography are steepening the base curve, increasing the lens diameter, and using a reverse geometry design. Because the patient already wears a relatively large diameter RGP lens with apical clearance and the lens is grossly decentered, a reverse geometry design was decided upon.

Fitting a reverse geometry design relies on diagnostic fitting. In most cases, a base curve slightly steeper than the postsurgical keratometry reading can be used.[1-4] If presurgical measurements are available, a base curve slightly flatter-than-K is a good starting point. The secondary or reverse curve is then made 3–7 diopters steeper than the base curve to align with the steeper mid-peripheral cornea.[2] The amount of steepening depends on the difference in curvature between the central and mid-peripheral corneas. Fitting sets can be borrowed from a local RGP lab to aid in this determination. In this case, a 3.00 D steeper secondary curve was selected. This design resulted in a well-centered lens with mild apical clearance and good mid-peripheral alignment. If the lens demonstrated excessive mid-peripheral and peripheral clearance, a steeper secondary curve could be ordered. The final lens should allow good positioning, movement, comfort, and vision.

Finally, thorough patient education on the visual outcomes is necessary. Even though this patient's glare symptoms were markedly reduced, he still noted some amount of glare, especially at night. However, he accepted that he will always see some glare and was happy we could reduce it.

Clinical Pearls

- Keratomileusis leaves a ring-shaped scar around the mid-periphery of the cornea.
- When fitting a post-refractive surgery cornea with RGP lenses, it is necessary to fit a large diameter or reverse geometry lens.
- Glare is a common symptom following refractive surgery and must be handled with thorough patient education and reassurance.

References

1. Chou A, Swinger CA, Cogger SK. Fitting contact lenses after myopic keratomileusis. *J Cataract Refract Surg.* 1999; 25(4):508–513.

2. Szczotka LB, Aronsky M. Contact lenses after LASIK. *J Am Optom Assoc.* 1998;69(12):775–784.
3. Stein HA, Harrison K. Contact lenses after refractive surgery. *Ophthalmol Clin North Am.* 1996;9(1):77–81.
4. Lim L, Siow K, Sakamoto R, et al. Reverse geometry contact lens wear after photorefractive keratectomy, radial keratotomy, or penetrating keratoplasty. *Cornea.* 2000;19(3):320–324.

Postsurgical Rigid Gas-Permeable Lens Intolerance

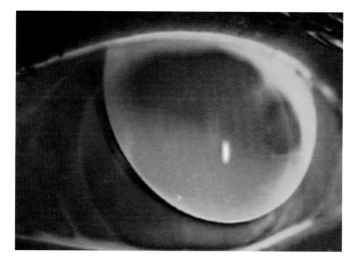

Figure 4-5

History

Patient RD, a 50-year-old Caucasian male, complains that his left contact lens (CL) is visually unstable and physically uncomfortable. His ocular history consists of two penetrating keratoplasty surgeries OS in 1970 and 1988 due to a chemical burn in 1970. He had cataract surgery with a PCIOL in 1985. In early 1999, he was fitted with spherical design rigid gas-permeable (RGP) contact lenses to correct his vision. He never adapted to the lens and presents in July 1999 with complaints of poor comfort, cloudy vision, and extensive mucous discharge.

Symptoms

- Poor RGP comfort
- Cloudy vision with RGP
- Mucous discharge

Clinical Data

- Entering visual acuity with spectacles:
  OD 20/20
  OS 20/400
- Subjective refraction:
  OD −3.50 sphere, 20/20
  OS −3.75 −2.00 × 120, 20/80
- Keratometry (from topography):
  OD 44.50 / 44.75 @ 090
  OS 48.83 @ 040 / 44.13 @ 160
- CL prescription OS: Boston ES 7.40 / −4.50 / 9.5, 20/40−
- CL fit OS: Superior temporal position, apical clearance, mid-peripheral bearing, excessive superior and inferior edge lift (see Figure 4-5)
- Biomicroscopy:
  OD Clear central corneal graft with few interrupted sutures, peripheral iridectomy, mild blepharitis
  OS Mild blepharitis, all other structures appear clear and healthy

Based on the clinical data, develop your list of differential diagnoses. Then, determine your final diagnosis and develop your treatment plan.

Differential Diagnoses

- Flat base curve
- High corneal toricity
- Graft tilt

Diagnosis

- Graft tilt with poorly fitting RGP
- Poor compliance with care regimen
- Blepharitis

Management

The patient experienced mucous discharge due to mild blepharitis, mild dry eye, and poor lens and lid hygiene. These problems were addressed before the lens was refit. A regimen of warm compresses, lid scrubs, and proper facial cleansing together with artificial tears alleviated symptoms of mucous discharge. The old contact lens was then assessed and found to be uncomfortable due to the excessive inferior edge lift. The fluorescein pattern was consistent with a vertically tilted graft due to the arcuate bearing along the superior graft margin. A new lens was ordered with a toric back surface to decrease the inferior edge lift. The new lens still maintained a superior position with arcuate bearing along the graft margin, but the patient reported very good comfort throughout his wearing time of 4–6 hours per day. Proper cleaning with the Boston Advance Comfort Formula and liquid enzyme maintain comfortable wear.

New CL prescription OS:

$$\text{Boston EO} \frac{7.40 / - 4.50}{6.90 / - 8.00} / 10.0 / 8.0 / \frac{8.90 @ 0.6/ 11.00 @ 0.4}{8.40 @ 0.6/ 10.50 @ 0.4} / 0.12$$

The patient currently wears his bitoric lens 4-6 hours per day with no problems. His visual acuity is 20/30+ with an over-refraction of plano −0.50 × 170, 20/25+. He is extremely happy with the comfort and vision with this lens. He returns for follow-up visits every 4 months.

Discussion

Penetrating keratoplasty commonly presents a challenge for postsurgical contact lens fitting due to corneal surface irregularities. In many cases, spherical-design RGP contact lenses are successful in providing a stable fit and vastly improved visual acuity. However, because of the large variations in postsurgical corneal topographies, alternate designs must sometimes be utilized.

Ideally, a normal topography of steep apex to flat periphery results after surgery. This topography usually can be successfully fit with spherical or aspheric RGP designs, and even soft lenses can be used if little corneal irregularity exists. However, soft lens wear is associated with higher rates of complications due to hypoxia, surface deposits, and tight lenses, and are generally not the lens of choice.[1-3]

When sufficient irregularity exists such that spherical RGP designs cannot be fit without visual, comfort, or ocular surface health compromises, specialty designs can be used. The shape and topography of the graft and host cornea must be considered when selecting the lens design. Fluorescein pattern assessment of a spherical RGP is valuable in helping determine a more appropriate design. The corneal shape irregularity can take on several forms due to variations in the graft:[4,5]

- Steep central topography due to a proud (large) graft
- Flat central topography due to tight sutures or a small graft
- Sloping topography due to a tilted or eccentric graft
- Irregular astigmatism due to variations in graft size or suturing technique

In many cases, these irregular topographies can be fit with spherical[1,2,4,6-10] or aspheric[11] RGP designs. Often, large diameter lenses are needed to achieve adequate centration and to vault the graft and minimize trauma. In cases where spherical designs fail due to poor fitting relationships, specialty lens designs may provide the patient with a stable, comfortable lens that offers visual improvement.[8,12-14] In these cases, computerized corneal topography has been invaluable in assisting the practitioner select the most appropriate RGP lens design.[15-17] Specialty designs that have been used include hybrid lenses, back and bitoric lenses, and reverse geometry designs.

Back-surface toric and bitoric designs are most useful when the postsurgical topography consists of large amounts of regular astigmatism. Since postsurgical astigmatism is often irregular, toric back surfaces usually are not indicated for the initial diagnostic lens. However, if fluorescein pattern evaluation reveals a highly toric pattern with resulting instability of lens fit, a toric back surface is indicated. Astigmatism, tilted grafts, or decentered grafts may require toric back-surface lenses.

This patient has a superiorly tilted graft that results in a cornea that is steep superiorly and flat inferiorly. A spherical back-surface lens has difficulty centering on this eye, and the sloping corneal surface causes excessive movement and edge lift in the vertical meridian. This results in discomfort and visual fluctuation. A toric back surface is fitted to lessen the edge lift in the vertical meridian and decrease movement. However, because the steepest area of the cornea is superior, the lens centers over this area. A decentered lens position is not ideal, but it can be acceptable provided the patient is comfortable and ocular surface health is not compromised. The selection of 3.50 D of toricity on the back surface is based on the corneal toricity (4.70 D, although irregular) and the appearance of the fluorescein pattern. The flat base curve is equal to the base curve of the old spherical lens. The steep base curve is made 3.50 D steeper than the flat base curve to reduce the inferior edge lift. The resulting fit is stable and provides good comfort and tear exchange.

The thought process behind the selection of specialty RGP designs must include an assessment of corneal topography and prior fluorescein pattern evaluation with a spherical RGP. Once this has been done, it is easier to determine the lens design that will improve the lens fit.

Clinical Pearls

- Post-penetrating keratoplasty corneal topography can take on several irregular shapes.
- Successful fitting of RGP lenses requires careful evaluation of the corneal topography and appropriate lens design selection.
- Tilted grafts can be fit with toric back-surface RGP designs when spherical designs fail.

References

1. Zadnik K. Post-surgical contact lens alternatives. *ICLC*. 1988; 15(7):211–219.
2. Moore JW. Contact lens fitting after penetrating keratoplasty. *Contact Lens Forum*. 1986;11(8):38–42.
3. Mannis MJ, Matsumoto ER. Extended-wear aphakic soft contact lenses after penetrating keratoplasty. *Arch Ophthalmol*. 1983; 101(8):1225–1228.
4. Caroline PJ, Zilge LB. Post-surgical correction with contact lens fitting following penetrating keratoplasty. In: Bennett ES, Weissman BA (eds). *Clinical Contact Lens Practice*. Philadelphia: J.B. Lippincott, 1992:Chapter 47, 1–14.
5. Philips AJ. Postkeratoplasty contact lens fitting. In: Harris MG (ed). *Contact Lenses for Pre- and Post-Surgery*. St. Louis: Mosby, 1997:97–131.
6. Beekhuis WH, van Rij G, Eggink FAGJ, et al. Contact lenses following keratoplasty. *CLAO J*. 1991;17(1):27–29.
7. Constad WH. Fitting post-op keratoplasty patients with RGP CLs. *Contact Lens Forum*. 1988;13(12):40–43.
8. Mannis MJ, Zadnik K, Deutch D. Rigid contact lens wear in the corneal transplant patient. *CLAO J*. 1986;12(1):39–42.
9. Manabe R, Matsuda M, Suda T. Photokeratoscopy in fitting contact lenses after penetrating keratoplasty. *Brit J Ophthalmol*. 1986;70(1):55–59.

10. Genvert GI, Cohen EJ, Arentsen JJ, Laibson PR. Fitting gas-permeable contact lenses after penetrating keratoplasty. *Am J Ophthalmol.* 1985;99(5):511–514.
11. Weiner BM, Nirankari VS. A new biaspheric contact lens for severe astigmatism following penetrating keratoplasty. *CLAO J.* 1992;18(1):29–33.
12. Metwalli MM. Meet the challenge of fitting the PKP cornea. *Review of Optom.* 1998;135(9):89–95.
13. Lindsay R. Post-keratoplasty contact lens management. *Clin Exp Optom.* 1995;78(6):223–226.
14. Binder PS, Kopecky L. Fitting the SoftPerm contact lens after keratoplasty. *CLAO J.* 1992;18(3):170–172.
15. Wicker D, Bleckinger P, Kowalski L, Wisniewski K. Gaining efficiency in fitting the post-penetrating keratoplasty patient. *Contact Lens Spectrum.* 1997;12(3):45–48.
16. Szczotka LB, Reinhart W. Computerized videokeratography contact lens software for RGP fitting in a bilateral postkeratoplasty patient: A clinical case report. *CLAO J.* 1995;21(1):52–56.
17. Lopatynsky M, Cohen EJ, Leavitt KG, Laibson PR. Corneal topography for rigid gas-permeable lens fitting after peneterating keratoplasty. *CLAO J.* 1993;19(1):41–44.

CASE 4-6

Uncomfortable Keratoconus Fit

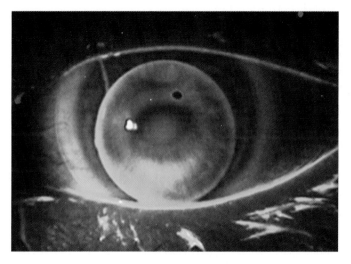

Figure 4-6

History

Patient AM, a 27-year-old Caucasian female, presents for her initial dispensing of a keratoconus rigid gas-permeable (RGP) contact lens (CL). The prior week, she was fit with a small, steep keratoconus design. Although the diagnostic lenses had fit with apical touch and mid-peripheral bubbles, the lens was ordered with a steeper base curve and flatter periphery to try to improve the fit. The ordered lens is not much better than the diagnostic lenses, with mild apical touch and mid-peripheral bubbles. This is the patient's first experience with contact lenses. Aside from the keratoconus, she has no ocular abnormalities. Her medical history is unremarkable, she takes no medications, and she has no known allergies.

Symptoms

Poor fit and comfort with her new keratoconus RGP lens

Clinical Data

- Entering visual acuity with spectacles:
  OD 20/15
  OS 20/800
- Spectacle prescription:
  OD Plano –0.50 × 054
  OS Plano –0.50 × 057
- Keratometry:
  OD 46.75 / 47.00 @ 100, clear mires
  OS >61.00 / 54.00 (corneal topographer unavailable)
- Subjective refraction:
  OD +0.25 –0.50 × 060, 20/15
  OS –4.00 sphere, 20/100
- Biomicroscopy:
  OD All structures clear and healthy
  OS Apical thinning and scarring, Vogt's striae, grade 1 apical staining
- Visual acuity with CL: OS 20/60
- Over-refraction OS: +1.00 –1.00 × 060, 20/40
- Fit assessment OS: Inferior position, good movement, apical touch, mid-peripheral clearance with bubbles, peripheral bearing with moderate edge lift (see Figure 4-6)
- CL prescription: Rose-K / 5.10 / –8.00 / 8.7 / 1.00 mm flat peripheral system

Based on the clinical data, develop your list of differential diagnoses. Then, determine your final diagnosis and develop your treatment plan.

Differential Diagnoses

- Flat base curve
- Steep peripheral curves
- Poor RGP candidate (keratoconus too severe)

Diagnosis

Poor fit with the current RGP design: too flat at apex, too steep in mid-periphery

Management

Because this patient was already fit with a very steep base curve and this particular clinic is very limited in its diagnostic lens choices for keratoconus, a piggyback system was attempted.

Soft lens: Frequency 55 / 8.4 / 14.2 / –0.75

The ordered Rose-K lens was placed on this soft lens. The fit was very steep, with central clearance and bubbles. Flatter lenses were subsequently tried over the soft lens. With a markedly flatter base curve, an alignment pattern was achieved centrally. The patient noted improved comfort and visual acuity with the piggyback system. The new RGP lens is

Rose-K / 6.00 / –1.75 / 8.7 / standard periphery
Visual acuity: 20/30
Fit assessment: Soft lens centered, 0.5 mm movement on blink
RGP centered, apical alignment, mild mid-peripheral clearance, moderate edge lift

The patient began wear of the piggyback system and was satisfied with the vision and comfort at her 1-week and 1-month follow-up visits. Apical staining was also reduced at her follow-up visits.

Discussion

Keratoconus can be a very challenging condition to manage with contact lenses. Mild cases can be fit fairly easily with either thick-design soft lenses or standard RGP designs. Moderate cases usually require a modified RGP design that is steeper centrally, flatter peripherally, and smaller in diameter. This is intended to more closely match the irregular corneal shape, so that the lens is stable and comfortable and provides good vision. Many RGP designs have been developed for keratoconus, including the Soper, McGuire, CLEK, and Rose-K designs. Although these designs work very well in many cases, there are times when they do not fit the eye satisfactorily. In such cases, alternate designs must be tried. When the keratoconus becomes severe, even the best RGP designs may not work for a given patient.

Alternative contact lens options for severe keratoconus include hybrid lenses, piggyback systems, and scleral lenses. Hybrid lenses (Soft-Perm) provide the best features of both soft and rigid lenses. The central portion is a low-Dk RGP that provides clear vision, while the peripheral portion is a low-water content soft lens that provides stability and comfort. It works quite well for patients who are intolerant to RGP lenses or when an RGP lens is unstable. In severe cases, it tends to fail because of a limited parameter range. In addition, the low-Dk value predisposes the patient to hypoxia-related complications, such as neovascularization. Therefore, for severe keratoconics, it is not the best option.

Scleral lenses are large-diameter lenses (20–25 mm) designed to vault the cornea and sit on the sclera. They have the advantage of eliminating the complexities of fitting the irregular corneal shape. However, they are not mainstream lenses and require expert fitting to provide good comfort and vision and prevent complications caused by poor tear exchange. For most, this option is a final one that just precedes referral for corneal transplant surgery.

Piggyback systems consist of a combination of soft and rigid lenses. First, a soft lens is placed on the cornea; then, an RGP lens is fit on top of it. The soft lens must center and demonstrate movement on blink. The RGP lens should align with the soft lens as closely as possible and also move slightly on a blink.[1-4] High-molecular-weight fluorescein is used to assess the fit of the RGP lens. This system provides the advantage of a smoother, flatter anterior ocular surface (the soft lens) that is easier to fit with an RGP. In addition, the decreased interaction of the RGP with the cornea and the decreased lens movement usually make patients more comfortable than wearing the RGP alone.[1-4] The disadvantages include the inconvenience of wearing and taking care of two different types of lenses and the decrease in oxygen transmissibility.[1-4] However, for severe keratoconics who cannot be fit with an RGP alone, it may prove to be a good option.

When selecting the soft lens, it should be a relatively high Dk/L design that drapes evenly over the cornea.[1-3] There should be no edge rippling, and the lens must move on the blink. A low minus power often is used because it provides a slightly flatter surface for the RGP fit. A plus power can be used if a more rounded surface is desired for fitting. Either way, the power of the soft lens is almost entirely neutralized by being sandwiched between the RGP and the cornea.

The RGP lens can then be fit on top of the soft lens. The fitting goals should be the same for an RGP alone: centration, moderate movement, apical alignment or light touch, mid-peripheral alignment, moderate peripheral clearance.[1-4]

Lens care can be confusing. Dispensing a system that is approved for both soft and rigid lenses, such as Solocare, often eliminates the confusion. Patient education on the reasons for fitting the piggyback system, symptoms of hypoxic and tight lens complications, and the necessity for regular follow-up is critical for long-term success. On follow-up visits, complications such as corneal edema, neovascularization, and acute red eye reactions must be detected early on. If the piggyback and other alternative contact lens systems fail, the patient may require an ophthalmological consult for a corneal transplant. However, with proper education and careful fitting and follow-up, severe keratoconus patients may enjoy years of comfortable, stable vision with a piggyback system.

Clinical Pearls

- Severe keratoconus may require alternative contact lens systems, such as a piggyback system.
- When fitting piggyback, select a soft lens that drapes evenly across the cornea. Then fit the RGP lens to the soft lens surface.
- Use high molecular weight fluorescein when evaluating the piggyback fit.
- Monitor the patient with a piggyback system carefully for signs of hypoxia-related complications.

References

1. Kok JHC, van Mil C. Piggyback lenses in keratoconus. *Cornea.* 1993;12(1):60–64.
2. Yeung K, Eghbali F, Weissman BA. Clinical experience with piggyback contact lens systems on keratoconic eyes. *J Am Optom Assoc.* 1995;66(9):539–543.
3. Tsubota K, Mashima Y, Murata H, Yamada M. A piggyback contact lens for the correction of irregular astigmatism in keratoconus. *Ophthalmol.* 1994;101(1):134–139.
4. Soper JW. Fitting keratoconus with piggyback and Saturn II lenses. *Contact Lens Forum.* 1986;11(8):25–30.

Orthokeratology, Part 1
Marjorie J. Rah

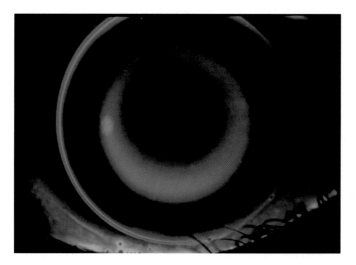

Figure 4-7

History

A 33-year-old Caucasian male presents to the clinic for the 1-day follow-up on his new orthokeratology contact lenses. The patient reports that the lenses are comfortable but his uncorrected vision is poor. During the baseline visit, the patient reported being active in swimming, biking, and running, during which he typically wears rigid gas-permeable (RGP) contact lenses (CL). He reported that RGP lenses were somewhat problematic while swimming due to the increased likelihood of losing a lens. He reported no personal history of medical problems but a family medical history of diabetes (maternal grandmother) and hypertension (mother). No known allergies to medications or environmental factors were reported, and the patient is not taking medication of any type.

Clinical Data

- Entering visual acuity with spectacles:
  OD 20/12.5
  OS 20/16
- Uncorrected visual acuity:
  OD 20/125
  OS 20/100
- Manifest refraction:
  OD –3.50 DS, 20/20
  OS –3.75 DS, 20/20
- Keratometry:
  OD 43.12 / 43.81 @ 090, smooth mires
  OS 43.50 / 43.94 @ 090, smooth mires
- Biomicroscopy: Unremarkable except for mild background papillary changes of the upper and lower tarsal conjunctiva in both eyes

Reverse geometry orthokeratology RGP contact lenses are ordered based on K-readings and refraction:

- Visual acuity with CL:
  OD 20/20
  OS 20/20
- CL fit assessment: Adequate central bearing zone (3–5 mm in diameter), adequate lens centration, adequate movement of lens (no lens binding), average edge lift OU (see Figure 4-7)
- Over-refraction:
  OD Plano sphere, 20/20
  OS –0.50 sphere, 20/20

At 1-day follow-up visit,

- Entering VA (with orthokeratology contact lenses):
  OD 20/15
  OS 20/15
- Uncorrected visual acuity:
  OD 20/50
  OS 20/40
- Manifest refraction:
  OD –2.25 –0.25 × 055, 20/20
  OS –2.00 –0.25 × 110, 20/20
- Keratometry:
  OD 41.17 / 42.06 @ 090 / smooth mires
  OS 41.75 / 42.37 @ 090 / smooth mires

- Biomicroscopy: Grade 1 conjunctival injection OU, grade 1 punctate fluorescein staining of the central, nasal, and temporal cornea OU

Based on the clinical data, determine the most appropriate course of action.

Differential Diagnoses

- Good initial orthokeratology response
- Poor initial orthokeratology response

Diagnosis

Good initial orthokeratology response

Management

After reassuring the patient that his uncorrected vision was not intended to be 20/20 on the first morning, he was asked to return approximately 8 hours later that day for a follow-up visit. At that time, uncorrected visual acuity was OD 20/80 and OS 20/60, and the refraction had regressed –0.50 D in the right eye and –0.75 D in the left. The patient was instructed to wear the lenses nightly for approximately 8–10 hours per night and return in 1 week for a follow-up appointment.

One week later, the patient reported that the lenses were quite comfortable and his uncorrected vision was very good. His uncorrected visual acuity was OD 20/15 and OS 20/15. Manifest refraction was OD +0.25 –0.25 × 085, 20/20, and OS +0.25 –0.50 × 090, 20/20. Keratometry had flattened to OD 40.00 / 40.62 @ 092 and OS 40.81 / 41.06 @ 092. Biomicroscopy revealed grade 1 punctate fluorescein staining of the nasal and temporal cornea OD, grade 1 punctate fluorescein staining of the central cornea OS, and grade 1.5 punctate fluorescein staining of the temporal cornea OS. That evening, his vision remained clear despite slight refractive regression.

The patient continued to have good vision and comfort at his 3-month and 1-year follow-up visits. At his 1-year follow-up visit, uncorrected visual acuity was OD 20/15 and OS 20/15. Manifest refraction was OD +0.25 –0.25 × 090, 20/15, and OS plano sphere, 20/15. Biomicroscopy revealed grade 1 corneal microcysts OU, grade 1 punctate fluorescein staining of the inferior cornea OD, grade 1 punctate fluorescein staining of the central cornea OS, grade 1 papillae of the lower tarsal conjunctiva OU, and grade 1 hyperemia of the upper palpebral conjunctiva OU.

Discussion

Orthokeratology is the application of RGP contact lenses designed to flatten the central cornea and temporarily reduce low to moderate amounts of myopic refractive error to improve unaided visual acuity. Traditional orthokeratology, popular in the 1970s and early 1980s, utilizes standard tricurve RGP contact lenses worn during waking hours. The technique consists of fitting a series of progressively flatter base curves, beginning approximately 0.25 to 0.75 diopters flatter than the flat keratometry reading.[1–3] Multiple lenses are necessary, each slightly flatter than the previous lens, until the desired treatment is achieved. Although this technique is safe, it is somewhat unpredictable and slow in achieving the desired treatment.[1,4,5] Another drawback is the limitation in the amount of myopia that can be corrected: 1–2 diopters.[6,7]

Interest in orthokeratology surged again with the introduction of reverse geometry RGP contact lenses designed for the procedure. This technique, known as accelerated orthokeratology, can be used to correct higher degrees of myopia (up to −6.00 diopters). Reverse geometry lenses classically are either three-curve or four-curve designs with a secondary curve radius that is steeper than the back optic zone radius. Presently, four-curve lens designs are used most commonly. These lenses consist of a back optic zone radius, a secondary curve that is steeper than the optic zone radius, an alignment zone radius, and a peripheral curve. The total diameter of the lenses typically ranges from 10.0–11.2 mm, which aids in better centering the lens on the eye. The optic zone diameter of this lens design usually is 6.0 mm.

Several reverse geometry lens designs currently are available for use in orthokeratology. Although each design has unique features, the fitting procedures are similar. The lenses can be worn either during waking hours or overnight. It is important to note that, as of this writing, overnight wear of reverse geometry lenses is not approved by the Food and Drug Administration.

When selecting patients for orthokeratology, the following issues should be considered. The patient must be motivated to wear the lenses and willing to agree to the necessary follow-up schedule. Orthokeratology is most successful for low to moderate amounts of myopia and with-the-rule astigmatism. It is not as successful for high myopia, high astigmatism, or moderate to high amounts of against-the-rule astigmatism. The patient must be motivated to wear the lenses and willing to comply with the rigorous follow-up visits. This, in combination with the previous diagnostic data, made him a suitable candidate for the procedure.

For the first 1–3 weeks of treatment, patients should expect variable vision throughout the day. The majority of changes in the corneal curvature occur during this period. Symptoms such as glare and halos may be reported. These symptoms should improve over time. Because they most likely are short-term effects, proper patient education is the best method of managing them. During the transition period, patients can wear their spectacles lenses (which will be overcorrected), wear hydrogel disposable lenses, or remain uncorrected (if the vision is adequate).

Patients who have never worn rigid lenses may have more difficulty adapting to orthokeratology lenses. Beginning with a traditional daily-wear rigid lens and switching to orthokeratology may help these patients gradually adapt to lens wear.

Also, during the first 1–3 weeks, most, if any, lens changes will be made. For this reason, regularly scheduled follow-up appointments are necessary. The importance of the 1-day visit is to assess the contact lens fit and evaluate the ocular health. The uncorrected visual acuity is not expected to be greatly improved at this time. Lens binding is not uncommon in orthokeratology and may be detected at this stage. The patient should be instructed on how to remove the lens if lens binding occurs. If lens binding becomes a chronic problem, the lens should be refitted. Some suggestions include using a contact lens material with a higher Dk value, decreasing the diameter of the lens, flattening the alignment or peripheral curve radius, and using artificial tears.[8]

Centration of the contact lens is a critical element in orthokeratology lens fitting. If the lens does not center well, the treatment zone on topography results in a steep change in curvature across the pupil. This most likely results in poor vision and induced astigmatism. It is important to fight the first instinct to make changes in the base curve. Changes in the alignment zone radius and overall diameter are necessary to provide better lens centration. For example, with high-riding or laterally decentered lenses, steepening the alignment zone radius or increasing the overall lens diameter may improve lens centration.[9]

Epithelial disruption with fluorescein staining of the cornea is common in patients undergoing overnight orthokeratology treatment. If corneal staining occurs, look for mechanical trauma or lack of tear exchange under the lens. A review of proper lens care is important to ensure the patient is compliant with lens cleaning and disinfecting. The addition of an enzymatic cleaner may aid in protein removal. If the problem persists, it may be necessary to refit the contact lens. Use of a lens material with a higher Dk may be necessary. In addition, modifying the peripheral curve of the lens may help to increase tear flow.

Clinical Pearls

- Accelerated orthokeratology utilizes reverse geometry RGP contact lenses and is indicated for myopia up to –6.00 D.
- Uncorrected vision is variable over the first 1–3 weeks.
- Lens centration is critical for good visual acuity.
- Lens binding and epithelial corneal staining may occur and must be managed accordingly.
- Patient education is important in managing patient compliance and in determining success in orthokeratology.

References

1. Mountford J. Orthokeratology. In: Philips AJ, Speedwell L (eds). *Contact Lenses*, 4th ed. Oxford: Butterworth–Heinemann, 1997:653–692.
2. Brand RJ, Polse KA, Schwalbe JS. The Berkeley Orthokeratology Study. Part I: General conduct of the study. *Am J Optom Physiol Opt.* 1983;60(3):175–186.
3. Kerns RL. Research in orthokeratology. Part II: Experimental design, protocol and method. *J Am Optom Assoc.* 1976; 47(10):1275–1285.
4. Hom MM. Orthokeratology Concepts. In: Hom MM (ed). *Manual of Contact Lens Prescribing and Fitting with* CD-ROM, 2nd ed. Boston: Butterworth–Heinemann, 2000:381–388.
5. Polse KA, Brand RJ, Keener RJ, et al. The Berkeley Orthokeratology Study. Part III: Safety. *Am J Optom Physiol Opt.* 1983; 60(4):321–328.
6. Polse KA, Brand RJ, Schwalbe JS, et al. The Berkeley Orthokeratology Study. Part II: Efficacy and duration. *Am J Optom Physiol Opt.* 1983;60(3):187–198.
7. Kerns RL. Research in orthokeratology. Part III: Results and observations. *J Am Optom Assoc.* 1976;47(12):1505–1515.

8. Hom MM, Watanabe R. Rigid gas-permeable cases. In: Hom MM (ed). *Manual of Contact Lens Prescribing and Fitting with CD-ROM*, 2nd ed. Boston: Butterworth–Heinemann, 2000:419–422.
9. Mountford J, Marsden HJ. Orthokeratology topography gallery. In: Hom MM (ed). *Manual of Contact Lens Prescribing and Fitting with CD-ROM*, 2nd ed. Boston: Butterworth–Heinemann, 2000:413–417.

CASE 4-8

Orthokeratology, Part 2

Harue J. Marsden

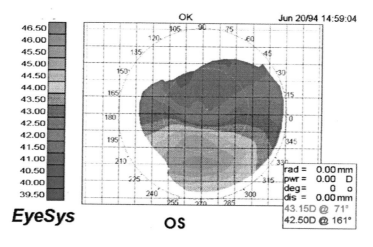

Figure 4-8

History

Patient BH, a 25-year-old Caucasian male, complains of blur at distance and monocular diplopia with the left eye through his spectacle correction. His medical history reveals orthokeratology contact lens wear for the past 8 months. His last eye exam was 8 months ago. He began wearing visual correction 10 years ago and has no significant ocular history. His last physical examination was 2 years ago, and he denies history of diabetes or cancer. He takes no medications. He reports an allergy to dust and pollen but has no known medication allergies. He has a family history of diabetes (maternal grandmother).

Symptoms

Monocular diplopia through his spectacle lenses; no diplopia noted with contact lens prescription

Clinical Data

- Refractive error prior to orthokeratology:
  OD –4.50 DS, 20/20
  OS –4.50 –0.25 × 90, 20/20
- Entering visual acuity with habitual spectacles:
  OD 20/20
  OS 20/20$^{-3/6}$
- Keratometry:
  OD 43.00 @ 90 / 42.50 @ 180, no distortion
  OS 44.00@60 / 43.00 @150, 1+ distortion
- Corneal topography: Reveals an area of inferior steepening, with an inferior minus superior (I – S) value of 3.50 D (see Figure 4-8)
- Refraction:
  OD –3.00 DS, 20/20
  OS –2.75 DS, 20/20$^{-2/6}$
- Biomicroscopy: 1+ blepharitis OU; 1+ conjunctival injection OU; corneas clear OU; anterior chamber deep and quiet OU; iris brown and homogeneous OU; lens clear OU
- Habitual contact lenses: Contex OK-3,
  OD 8.70 mm / –1.00 D / 10.0 mm / 6.0 mm / SC 8.08 mm; VA 20/20
  OS 8.60 mm / –0.50 D / 10.0 mm / 6.0 mm / SC 7.99 mm; VA 20/20
- Over-refraction:
  OD +0.25 DS, 20/20
  OS: +0.25 –0.50 × 080, 20/20
- Fluorescein pattern:
  OD Apical touch/no toricity/good mid-peripheral pooling/centered
  OS Apical touch/no toricity/good mid-peripheral pooling/superior position

Develop your list of differential diagnoses. Then, based on the clinical data, determine your final diagnosis. Based on your diagnosis, develop your treatment plan.

Differential Diagnoses

- Keratoconus
- Inferior apical displacement (corneal warpage) secondary to a high-riding, flat-fitting rigid contact lens

Diagnosis

Inferior apical displacement (corneal warpage) secondary to high-riding, flat-fitting rigid contact lens

Management

You decide that your options are

1. Rigid gas-permeable (RGP) contact lenses refit to achieve an interpalpebral, centered contact lens design
2. Maintain lid-attachment flat-fitting rigid contact lens fit
3. Refit with a hydrogel lens design
4. Discontinue all lens wear

BH was refit on the same day. A steeper-fitting, conventional tricurve lens design was used to improve lens centration. The initial diagnostic lens was selected using the patient's average keratometry readings less 1.25 D to create an approximate tear lens of –1.25 D. These contact lens parameters give a lens fit approximately 0.50 D flatter than an alignment contact lens fit. Contact lenses prescribed: FluoroPerm 30,

OD 8.00 mm / –2.00 D / 10.5 mm / 9.0 mm / 8.70 mm / 1.5 pd; VA 20/20
OS 7.99 mm / –2.25 D / 10.5 mm / 9.0 mm / 8.69 mm / 1.5 pd; VA 20/20

Prism was ordered to improve lens centration. The patient returned in 1 week so that the contact lenses could be dispensed.

- Entering visual acuity:
  OD 20/20
  OS 20/20
- Over-refraction:
  OD +0.25 DS, $20/20^{+2/6}$
  OS +0.25 –0.25 × 090, $20/20^{+3/6}$

- Fluorescein pattern:
  OD Slight apical touch/no toricity/average edge clearance/ centered
  OS Slight apical touch/no toricity/average edge clearance/ centered

The patient returned to the clinic 1 week after receiving the conventional rigid gas-permeable contact lens. Four months after the refit, BH reports full-time wearing of his RGP lenses and elimination of the monocular diplopia.

- Entering visual acuity at distance:
  OD 20/20
  OS 20/20
  OU 20/20
- Corneal topography: A symmetrical, spherical pattern with an inferior minus superior (I − S) value of 1.00 D
- Refraction:
  OD −4.00 DS, 20/20
  OS −3.75 DS, 20/20

Discussion

BH demonstrates the corneal topographical changes often found in lid attachment or superior positioning, flat-fitting RGP contact lenses. These have been described as "pseudokeratoconus," and some researchers have speculated that this type of lens fit may lead to keratoconus. BH has no slit-lamp findings of Vogt's striae, Fleischer ring, or corneal thinning. Although his corneal topography exhibited an I − S value of 3.50 D, which is suspicious of keratoconus,[1] in the absence of any slit-lamp findings, it was determined that BH was not keratoconic.

During the orthokeratology treatment phase, BH initially was fit with a reverse geometry rigid contact lens with a base curve approximately 2.00 D flatter than his flat keratometry measurement. Subsequent lenses were fit flatter to further enhance the orthokeratology effect. Following 8 months of orthokeratology, the base curve of the left contact lens was approximately 4.00 D flatter than the initial base curve. The contact lens positioned superiorly, and as a result, the corneal apex is displaced inferiorly. Superior positioning orthokeratology lenses can induce unwanted astigmatism.[2,3] The complaint of monocular diplopia is a consequence of 3.00 D of corneal power differences on the visual axis.

Using steeper-fitting reverse geometry rigid contact lenses did not improve centration, so steeper-fitting conventional RGP contact lenses are diagnostically fit. Large overall diameter RGP lenses with 1.5 diopters of prism are prescribed to improve lens centration. With improved centration, the corneal distortion is alleviated resulting in symmetrical corneal topography. Unfortunately, the orthokeratology effect is diminished as a result of refitting. The initial decrease of the orthokeratology is approximately 2.00 D of myopia. Following the refit, the decrease in myopia from baseline is nearly 1.00 D. The patient is satisfied with the outcome and continues to wear conventional tri-curve RGP lenses. With the spherical, uniform corneal topography, the diameter has been decreased from 10.5 mm to 10.0 mm and prism no longer is prescribed in the contact lenses.

Corneal sphericalization may occur following orthokeratology.[4] Topographical changes should reveal a smooth, uniform curvature over the corneal surface. Reverse-geometry lenses may yield more aggressive results, including larger magnitudes of myopia reduction. The topographical outcome resembles an oblate surface similar to a post-refractive-surgery cornea. Similar symptomatology of haloes, ghost images, and glare may accompany these topographical changes. Patient education regarding realistic expectations of visual side effects is imperative. Lens centration is critical for optimal orthokeratology results.

Clinical Pearls

- Lens centration is critical for successful orthokeratology treatment.
- Steeper base curves, larger overall diameters, and prism ballast may help center a superior positioning RGP lens.
- Superior positioning reverse-geometry orthokeratology lenses may need refitting to conventional RGP designs.
- The topographical outcome of successful orthokeratology is an oblate surface similar to a post-refractive-surgery cornea, with similar potential symptomatology of haloes, ghost images, and glare. Patient education regarding the visual side effects is imperative for informed consent of orthokeratology candidates.

References

1. Rabinowitz YS, McDonnell PJ. Computer assisted corneal topography in keratoconus. *Refract Corneal Surg.* 1989;5(6):400–408.
2. Kerns RL. Research in orthokeratology Part III: Results and observations. *J Am Optom Assoc.* 1976;47(12):1505–1515.
3. Kerns RL. Research in orthokeratology Part IV: Results and observations. *J Am Optom Assoc.* 1977;48(2):227–238.

4. Woo GC, Chow E, Cheng D, Woo S. A study of the central and peripheral refractive power of the cornea with orthokeratology treatment. *Int Contact Lens Clin*. 1994;21(7):132–135.

Occluder Pupil Lens and a Red Eye

Nadia S. Zalatimo

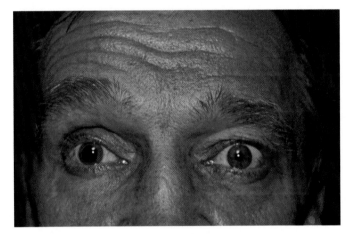

Figure 4-9

History

A 49-year-old Caucasian male presents for examination with complaints of reduced vision and glare OD, causing visual discomfort. The patient reports glare, worse in bright lighting conditions, and difficulty driving at night. He has no complaints with his vision OS. The patient reports a history of traumatic retinal detachment 3 years ago OD, treated with lensectomy and scleral buckle procedures. Subsequently, the patient developed proliferative vitreoretinopathy, which necessitated implantation of silicon oil, which later was removed. The patient's left eye is status post laser photocoagulation for an atrophic retinal hole 2 years prior. The patient reports contact lens wear in the past with no complications. The patient's medical history is significant for chronic hepatitis C and post-traumatic stress disorder. The patient is taking no medications and has no known medical allergies.

Symptoms

Glare OD, especially in bright light conditions

Clinical Data

- Entering visual acuity at distance with habitual prescription:
  OD 4/700
  OS 20/20
- Entering visual acuity at near OS: 20/25
- Extraocular motility: Smooth, accurate, full, extensive in all fields of gaze
- Confrontation fields:
  OD Constricted 360° to facial field
  OS Full to finger counting
- Pupils:
  OD 4 mm in light, 5 mm in dark
  OS 3 mm in light, 4 mm in dark
  Trace reactive OD, 3+ reactive OS, +APD OD
- Habitual spectacle prescription:
  OD −1.75 −0.25 × 156
  OS −1.75 −0.25 × 144
  Add +1.50
- Manifest refraction:
  OD +12.50, 20/300
  OS −1.75 −0.25 × 144, 20/20
  Add +1.75, 20/20 OS
- Keratometry:
  OD 39.75/41.00 @ 091
  OS 40.50/40.75 @ 046, mires clear and regular on
- Biomicrosopy: Vitreous prolapse and Iridodonesis OD; otherwise, all structures appear clear and healthy
- Goldmann applanation tonometry: 17 mm Hg OD, 18 mm Hg OS @ 2:00 P.M.
- Dilated fundus examination:
  Lens: Aphakia OD, clear OS
  Optic nerve: 0.7 with diffuse atrophy OD, 0.8 with healthy rim OS

Macula: Flat OU with retinal pigmented epithelium (RPE) migration OD
Periphery: Retinal attached on scleral buckle 360° OD; flat and intact with laser scarring surrounding atrophic hole at 8:00 OS

Differential Diagnosis

- Uncorrected aphakia
- Anisocoria with permanently reduced visual acuity OD
- Corneal edema

Diagnosis

Anisocoria with permanently reduced visual acuity OD

Management

The patient's right eye was fit with an opaque pupil contact lens to block light entering the pupil and eliminate symptoms of glare: in-office trial 1, WJ Durasoft 3 / 8.6/14.5 / 4 mm Occluder pupil. This lens provided complete corneal coverage and good movement (0.5 mm), but the patient reported persistence of glare around the edges of the pupil: in-office trial 2, WJ Durasoft 3 / 8.6/14.5 / 6 mm Occluder pupil. This lens provided complete corneal coverage, good movement (0.5 mm), and full pupil coverage with significant reduction of glare symptoms OD. The lens was dispensed to the patient with proper instructions on lens care. The patient was advised to return for follow-up within 2 weeks.

At the 2-week follow-up examination, the patient reported increased comfort in bright light conditions with contact lens wear but still noticed glare from the nasal field. He stated that the residual glare created persistent difficulty driving at night, so he wanted a darker pupil. The patient also complained that the lens felt dry and uncomfortable by the end of the day. Average wearing time was 13 hours. Biomicroscopy found the following:

- Contact lens fit: Minimal movement, tears trapped beneath lens; lens centered, no adhesion
- Conjunctiva: 1+ diffuse injection around limbus OD, clear OS
- Cornea: +central superficial punctate keratitis (SPK) OD, clear OS

The patient had a tight fit causing SPK due to minimal tear exchange and symptoms of discomfort after prolonged wear. The opaque pupil was not large enough or dark enough, causing persistent complaints of glare.

The patient was refit with a flatter base curve to improve movement. The opaque pupil was enlarged to 6.5 mm, and the darkness of opaque pupil increased: in-office trial 3, Coopervision Hydrasoft / 9.2 / plano / 15.0. The lens demonstrated good centration, coverage, and movement. The patient reported good comfort. The lens was sent to Adventures in Color to provide a 6.5 mm black opaque pupil, then dispensed with proper instructions on lens care using a hydrogen peroxide cleaning and disinfecting regimen. The patient was instructed to return in 2 weeks for follow-up examination.

At the next 2-week follow-up examination, the patient reported he was very happy with the contact lens. He was much more comfortable in bright light conditions, noticed no glare, and had no difficulty driving at night. He stated that the lens was comfortable, and he noticed no irritation. He reported using nonpreserved artificial tears bid-qid for dryness but had no other complaints. Biomicroscopy revealed the following:

- Contact lens fit: Good centration, movement, coverage (see Figure 4-9)
- Conjunctiva: Trace injection OD, clear OS
- Cornea: Clear OU, no SPK OD

The new lens fit was acceptable, and dry eye was controlled with nonpreserved tears. A 1-month follow-up was recommended.

The patient returned 4 months later for a contact lens follow-up examination, complaining of a red, irritated eye OD for 2 days. He noted intermittent irritation and itching over the past month, which would improve with cessation of lens wear for 1–2 days. He also reported tearing, itching, and a swollen eyelid, which worsened progressively over the preceding 2 days. The patient stated that he wore the lens an average of 14 hours daily, stored the lens in ReNu multipurpose solution, and used Supraclens twice a week. The patient did not digitally clean the lens. He used nonpreserved artificial tears only when the eyes felt irritated. The patient had not worn the lens since the night before but brought it with him. Biomicroscopy revealed the following:

- Lids: + erythematous, mildly edematous upper lid OD, clear OS

- Conjunctiva: 2+ follicles on upper palpebral conjunctiva, 3+ follicles on lower palpebral conjunctiva, 1+ diffuse injection OD, clear OS
- Cornea: Moderately dense diffuse SPK OD, trace SPK OS; no edema OU
- Contact lens evaluation: Diffuse protein deposits

Your differential diagnosis of these signs is:

- Contact lens overwear syndrome
- Giant papillary conjunctivitis
- Allergic keratoconjunctivitis
- Toxic keratoconjunctivitis
- Infectious keratitis
- Dry eye
- Mechanical trauma

Diagnosis

The patient has allergic keratoconjunctivitis caused by contact lens solutions. Lens wear was discontinued until the eye was quiet. Nonpreserved artificial tears were prescribed q2h during waking hours. The patient was reeducated to use only hydrogen peroxide solutions for cleaning and disinfecting his contact lens, and the importance of digital rubbing was stressed. The allergic conjunctivitis resolved within a few weeks, and the patient successfully returned to full-time wear, using a hydrogen peroxide care system.

Discussion

Glare from a nonseeing eye can cause difficulty functioning in bright light and glare conditions and can negatively affect one's quality of life. Glare can be effectively eliminated with the use of occluder pupil contact lenses.[1] Occluder or opaque pupil contact lenses can be ordered directly through certain contact lens manufacturers. Another option is to have an opaque pupil added to a clear hydrogel contact lens by a specialty contact lens tinting company. The advantage to adding a pupil to a clear lens is that the opaque pupil can be made darker and the size of the opaque pupil can be specifically requested.

When fitting an opaque pupil contact lens, it is important to first ensure that the lens fits well. The addition of tint to a lens can produce a thicker, stiffer, heavier lens that has lower oxygen transmissibility.[2] It is important to consider this when fitting the lens and to choose the flattest base curve that provides an acceptable fit.[3] The next step is to determine the size of opaque pupil desired. It is important to consider pupil size in the dark. For maximal occlusion, the opaque pupil size should be slightly larger than the dark pupil size. In this case, the patient complained of peripheral glare that caused difficulty driving at night. Increasing the diameter of the pupil size relieved the symptoms. Although cosmetically noticeable, the larger diameter provided symptomatic relief from glare and was preferable to the patient.

Patients wearing cosmetic lenses should be educated on the importance of proper lens care and follow up. Such patients are prone to contact lens overwear, since they depend on their lens for visual or emotional comfort and often are reluctant to remove the lens despite discomfort. In addition, some chemical solutions can cause the tint to fade, and it is recommended that the lens manufacturer be consulted as to the ideal disinfecting system.[4]

In this case, the patient developed allergic conjunctivitis due to a delayed hypersensitivity reaction to the multipurpose disinfection solution. The patient had switched from a hydrogen peroxide disinfecting system to a multipurpose solution because of ease of cleaning. Although contact lens–associated red eye can have many causes, several factors in this case are consistent with allergic conjunctivitis. The fact that the patient's symptoms of itching, irritation and redness resolved with cessation of lens wear and became worse with longer wearing time points to the lens or the solutions as the cause. Examination showed follicles and conjunctival hyperemia, which are signs of allergy, with no sign of corneal hypoxia or trauma, such as infiltrates, edema, or abrasion. Dense, diffuse superficial punctate keratitis was present but was attributed to keratitis sicca, which is consistent with his history of dry eye, the presence of SPK in the fellow eye, and poor compliance with his artificial tears. A toxic chemical reaction was ruled out because the redness, irritation and SPK did not occur immediately after application of the lens to the eye, which is the typical response.[5] Allergic conjunctivitis caused by contact lens solutions typically is a delayed hypersensitivity response that occurs after several months of repeated and prolonged exposure to the offending chemical.

Cosmetic contact lenses can significantly enhance the quality of life in patients suffering from visual discomfort or disfigurement. Care should be taken to achieve a good fit and educate the patient extensively on proper lens care and follow-up to avoid contact lens–related complications.

Clinical Pearls

- Symptomatic glare from a nonseeing eye can be successfully managed with an occluder contact lens.
- To achieve the darkest occlusion, have the opaque pupil added to well-fitting hydrogel lens.
- Always check the fit of the clear lens before having the opaque pupil added.
- Use the flattest lens possible while maintaining an acceptable fit.
- Consult the lens manufacturer for proper disinfecting solutions to avoid fading.
- Measure pupil size in the dark to avoid peripheral glare from too small occluder pupil size.

References

1. Scott C, White P. Contact lens care and supplemental procedures. *Contact Lens Spectrum.* 1996;11(11):42–47.
2. Wodak G. Soft artificial iris lenses. *Contact.* November 1977; 21:4–8.
3. Shovlin J, Meshel L, et al. Tinted contact lenses: Cosmetic and prosthetic application. In: Bennett ES, Weissman BA (eds). *Clinical Contact Lens Practice.* Philadelphia: J.B. Lippincott, 1992:Chapter 52, 1–8.
4. Cassel M. Twelve steps to successful prosthetic soft contact lens fitting. *Contact Lens Spectrum.* 1996;11(12):20-21, 23–25.
5. Caffery BE, Josephson, JE. Complications of lens care solutions. In: Silbert JA (ed). *Anterior Segment Complications of Contact Lens Wear,* 2nd ed. Boston: Butterworth–Heinemann, 2000:149–163.

Index

adherence, keratoconus and, 173–178
adhesion, 159–164
against-the-rule corneas, laterally decentered lens and, 9–13
allergic keratoconjunctivitis, 224–225, 226
aniscoria, 221–227
aspheric lenses, visual flare and, 50–55
astigmatism
    flexure and, 70–71
    orthokeratology and, 207–220
    pellucid marginal corneal degeneration and, 186–188
    soft versus rigid toric lenses and, 35–38
axis location with toric soft lens, 31–32

base curves
    aspheric lenses and, 53–54
    blurry, uncomfortable soft lens and, 25–28
    keratoconus and uncomfortable fit, 201–205
    low-riding lens and, 6
    orthokeratology and, 218–219
    unstable bitoric lens and, 41–42
bifocal lenses, 179–183
bitoric lenses, 36–38
    base curve selection for, 41–42
    flexure and, 66–71
    high-riding lens and, 16–18
    peripheral curves and, 42
    postsurgical, 198
    power determination for, 42–43
    unstable, 39–43
blepharitis, 85–87, 133–137, 195–200
blink characteristics
    low-riding lenses and, 5
    slow post-blink return and, 32

care systems. *See also* preservative sensitivity
    alcohol-based, 85–86
    allergic keratoconjunctivitis from, 224–225, 226
    CLARE and, 165–169
    foggy vision with, 83–87
    giant papillary conjunctivitis and, 136
    infiltrates from, 143–146
    lens contamination and, 81–82
    poor adherence to, 195–200
    selection of, 64
    thimerosal in, 141–142
center thickness, low-riding lens and, 6–7
centration
    aspheric lenses and, 53–54
    lens adhesion and, 162–163
    orthokeratology and, 211–212, 217, 218–219
    RGP postsurgical, 189–193
    visual flare and, 47–50
cleaning lenses, excessive, 63–65
cloudy vision, 79–82
conjunctivitis, 120. *See also* red eye
    allergic keratoconjunctivitis, 224–225, 226
    giant papillary, 127–131, 133–137
contact lens acute red eye (CLARE), 104, 165–169
corneal cylinder undercorrection, 39–43
corneal desiccation, low-riding lens and, 3–8
corneal sphericalization, 219
corneal ulcers, 147–151
    microbial, 153–158
    sterile versus infectious, 149–150
corneal warpage, 216–220
    double vision and, 73–77

corneas
    against-the-rule, 9–13
    with-the-rule, high-riding lens and,
        16–18

desiccation
    rigid lens, 117–126
    soft lens, 111–115, 117–126
discomfort
    CLARE and, 165–169
    high-riding lens and, 15–18
    laterally decentered lens and, 9–13
    lens desiccation and, 117–126
    low-riding lens and, 3–8, 19–23
    with RGPs, 159–164
    with soft lenses, 111–115, 139–142,
        153–158
disposable lenses, 129, 130
dry eyes
    causes of, 113
    foggy vision and, 83–87
    lens contamination and, 81–82
    lens desiccation and, 111–115
    punctal occlusion and, 120–121
    vascularized limbal keratitis and,
        123–126

edge design
    giant papillary conjunctivitis and, 136
    laterally decentered lens and, 9–13
    low-riding lens and, 7
episcleritis, 141
epithelial splitting, 107–110
eyelid anatomy
    epithelial splitting and, 107–110
    foggy vision and, 83–87
    improving attachment and, 22–23
    low-riding lens and, 7, 19–23
    RGP fit and, 185–188
    tight, 19–23

fit-induced complications
    discomfort with soft lenses, 111–115,
        139–142, 153–158
    infiltrates, 143–146
    itchy RGP lenses, 132–137
    itchy soft lenses, 127–131
    pain with soft lenses, 107–110,
        165–169

redness with RGPs, 117–126
    redness with soft lenses, 101–105,
        153–158, 165–169
    RGP discomfort, 159–164
    white spots, 147–151
fitting problems
    blurry, uncomfortable soft lens, 25–28
    high-riding lens, 15–18
    laterally decentered lens, 9–13
    low-riding lens, 3–8, 19–23
    poor vision with toric soft lens, 29–33
    of soft versus rigid toric lenses, 35–38
    unstable bitoric lenses, 39–43
flat lenses
    high-riding, 16–18
    laterally decentered, 9–13
    low-riding, 3–8
    orthokeratology and, 216–220
    soft toric, 32
flexure, 66–71
foggy vision, 83–87

giant papillary conjunctivitis (GPC),
        127–131
    RGP lens–induced, 133–137
glare. *See also* visual flare
    occluder pupil lens and, 221–227
    postsurgical, 189–193

hole-in-the-hand test, 90–91
hybrid lenses, 204
hypoxia, 27, 145–146

inferior position, low-riding lenses and,
        5–8
infiltrates, 143–146
    CLARE and, 167
interpalpebral fit, low-riding lens and,
        22–23
itchy lenses
    RGP, 132–137
    soft, 127–131

keratoconus, 120
    pellucid marginal corneal degeneration
        versus, 187–188
    pseudokeratoconus and, 73–77
    uncomfortable RGP in, 173–178,
        201–205

keratomileusis, 189–193
keratoplasty, 195–200

lens diameter
    laterally decentered lens and, 12
    low-riding lens and, 6
lens movement, unstable bitoric lens and,
    39–43
lens rotation, with toric soft lens, 29–33
lesions
    corneal ulcers, 147–151, 153–158
    superior epithelial arcuate, 107–110
    vascularized limbal keratitis, 123–126

makeup contamination, 79–82
marginal degeneration, 185–188
meibomitis, 83–87
microbial corneal ulcers, 153–158
modulus determination, 70–71
monovision, 90–93, 96–97
    bifocal lenses versus, 179–183
mucous discharge, 153–158, 195–200
    giant papillary conjunctivitis and,
        127–131
multifocal lenses
    alternating design, 179–183
    bifocal lenses versus, 179–183
    presbyopia and, 96–98

nonwetting, foggy vision and, 83–87. *See
    also* dry eyes

occluder pupil lenses, 221–227
optical cross, for bitoric lenses, 42–43
optical problems
    blurry near vision, 89–98
    blurry vision, 61–71
    cloudy vision, 79–82
    double vision, 73–77
    foggy vision, 83–87
    sudden onset blur, 57–60
    visual flare, 47–55
optic zone diameter, visual flare and,
    47–50
orthokeratology, 207–220
overcleaning, 63–65

patient history, 155–156
pellucid marginal degeneration, 185–188
peripheral curve design
    for bitoric lenses, 42

low-riding lens and, 7
photophobia, 153–158
piggyback lenses, 204–205
postsurgical glare, 189–193
presbyopia, 89–98
    bifocal lenses and, 179–183
    monovision and, 90–93, 96–97,
        179–183
preservative sensitivity, 5, 103–104
    infiltrates from, 143–146
    laterally decentered lens and, 11
    lens desiccation and, 114
pseudokeratoconus, 73–77, 162, 218
punctal occlusion, 114, 120–121

red eye
    causes of, 103–104
    CLARE and, 165–169
    low-riding lens and, 3–8
    occluder pupil lens and, 221–227
    with RGPs, 117–126
    with soft lens, 101–105, 153–158
    superior limbic keratoconjunctivitis,
        139–142
reverse geometry lenses, 207–220
rigid gas-permeable lenses (RGPs)
    adherence of, 173–178
    adhesion, 159–164
    bifocal, 179–183
    blurry vision with rigid, 61–71
    care system selection for, 64
    cloudy vision with, 79–82
    desiccation of, 117–126
    difficult fit, 185–188
    discomfort with, 159–164
    flexure of, 66–71
    foggy vision with, 83–87
    giant papillary conjunctivitis and,
        133–137
    high-riding, 15–18
    itchy, 133–137
    keratoconus and uncomfortable,
        173–178, 201–205
    laterally decentered, 9–13
    low-riding, 3–8, 19–23
    orthokeratology and, 207–220
    overcleaning, 63–65
    postsurgical glare with, 189–193
    postsurgical intolerance of, 195–200
    redness with, 117–126
    sudden onset blur with, 57–60

rigid gas-permeable lenses, *cont.*
  surface contamination of, 79–82
  unstable bitoric, 39–43
  visual flare with, 47–55

scleral lenses, 204
sighting dominance, 90–91
soft lens–associated chronic hypoxia
    (SLACH), 104, 167
soft lenses
  blurry, uncomfortable, 25–28
  CLARE and, 165–169
  desiccation of, 111–115
  discomfort with, 111–115, 139–142
  infiltrates from, 143–146
  itchy, 127–131
  keratoconus and, 204–205
  microbial corneal ulcers and, 153–158
  pain with, 107–110, 153–158,
     165–169
  redness with, 101–105, 153–158,
     165–169
  tight-fitting, 101–105
specialty lens fitting dilemmas
  bifocal, 179–183
  difficult RGP fit, 185–188
  occluder pupil lens, 221–227
  orthokeratology, 207–220
  postsurgical glare, 189–193
  postsurgical RGP intolerance, 195–200
  uncomfortable keratoconus, 201–205
  uncomfortable RGP in keratoconus,
    173–178
staining, 3 and 9 o'clock, 6, 119–120
  vascularized limbal keratitis and, 125
steep lenses
  blurry, uncomfortable soft, 25–28
  detecting, 27
  laterally decentered, 9–13
  low-riding, 3–8
  soft toric, 32–33
steroids, 145–146
superficial punctate keratitis (SPK),
    224–225
superior epithelial arcuate lesions
    (SEALs), 107–110
superior limbic keratoconjunctivitis
    (SLK), 139–142

surface contamination, 79–82
  foggy vision with, 83–87
  giant papillary conjunctivitis and, 129
surgery
  glare after, 189–193
  RGP intolerance after, 195–200
switched lenses, 57–60

tarsal papillary hypertrophy, 129
thimerosal, 141–142
toric lenses
  back-surface, 198–199
  double vision with, 73–77
  laterally decentered, 12
  poor vision with soft, 29–33
  postsurgery, 198
  soft versus rigid, 35–38

ulcers, corneal, 147–151
  microbial, 153–158
  sterile versus infectious, 149–150

vascularized limbal keratitis (VLK),
    123–126
videokeratography, 187, 188
visual acuity
  bifocal lenses and, 179–183
  blur rejection and, 36–38
  blurry
    uncomfortable soft lens and, 25–28
    with RGPs, 61–71
  blurry near vision, 89–98
  cloudy vision, 79–82
  double vision, 73–77
  foggy vision, 83–87
  orthokeratology and, 207–220
  poor, with toric soft lens, 29–33
  of soft versus rigid toric lenses, 35–38
  sudden onset blur, 57–60
  unstable bitoric lens and, 39–43
visual flare, 47–55
  aspheric lenses and, 51–55
  occluder pupil lens and, 221–227
  postsurgical, 189–193

wear time, excessive, 101–105
  CLARE and, 165–169
white spots, 147–151